CARDIOLOGY RESEARCH AND CLINICAL DEVELOPMENTS SERIES:

CARDIOVASCULAR SIGNALS IN DIABETES MELLITUS: A NEW TOOL TO DETECT AUTONOMIC NEUROPATHY

CARDIOLOGY RESEARCH AND CLINICAL DEVELOPMENTS SERIES

Focus on Atherosclerosis Research
Leon V. Clark (Editor)
2004. ISBN: 1-59454-044-6

Cholesterol in Atherosclerosis and Coronary Heart Disease
Jean P. Kovala (Editor)
2005. ISBN: 1-59454-302-X

Frontiers in Atherosclerosis Research
Karin F. Kepper (Editor)
2007. ISBN: 1-60021-371-5

Cardiac Arrhythmia Research Advances
Lynn A. Vespry (Editor)
2007. ISBN: 1-60021-794-X

Cardiac Arrhythmia Research Advances
Lynn A. Vespry (Editor)
2007. ISBN: 978-1-60692-539-3
(Online Book)

Heart Disease in Women
Benjamin V. Lardner and Harrison R. Pennelton (Editors)
2009. ISBN: 978-1-60692-066-4

Heart Disease in Women
Benjamin V. Lardner and Harrison R. Pennelton (Editors)
2010. ISBN: 978-1-60741-090-4 (Online Book)

Cardiomyopathies: Causes, Effects and Treatment
Peter H. Bruno and Matthew T. Giordano (Editors)
2009. ISBN: 978-1-60692-193-7

Cardiomyopathies: Causes, Effects and Treatment
Peter H. Bruno and Matthew T. Giordano (Editors)
2009. ISBN: 978-1-60876-433-4 (Online Book)

Transcatheter Coil Embolization of Visceral Arterial Aneurysms
Shigeo Takebayashi, Izumi Torimoto and Kiyotaka Imoto (Editors)
2009. ISBN: 978-1-60741-439-1

Transcatheter Coil Embolization of Visceral Arterial Aneurysms
Shigeo Takebayashi, Izumi Torimoto and Kiyotaka Imoto (Editors)
2009. ISBN: 978-1-978-1-60876-797-7
(Online Book)

Heart Disease in Men
Alice B. Todd and Margo H. Mosley (Editors)
2009. ISBN: 978-1-60692-297-2

Angina Pectoris: Etiology, Pathogenesis and Treatment
Alice P. Gallos and Margaret L. Jones (Editors)
2009. ISBN: 978-1-60456-674-1

Coronary Artery Bypasses
Russell T. Hammond and James B Alton (Editors)
2009. ISBN: 978-1-60741-064-5

Congenital Heart Defects: Etiology, Diagnosis and Treatment
Hiroto Nakamura (Editor)
2009. ISBN: 978-1-60692-559-1

Congenital Heart Defects: Etiology, Diagnosis and Treatment
Hiroto Nakamura (Editor)
2009. ISBN: 978-1-60876-434-1 (Online Book))

Atherosclerosis: Understanding Pathogenesis and Challenge for Treatment
Slavica Mitrovska, Silvana Jovanova Inge Matthiesen and Christian Libermans
2009. ISBN: 978-1-60692-677-2

Practical Rapid ECG Interpretation (PREI)
Abraham G. Kocheril and Ali A. Sovari
2009. ISBN: 978-1-60741-021-8

Heart Transplantation: Indications and Contraindications, Procedures and Complications
Catherine T. Fleming (Editor)
2009. ISBN 978-1-60741-228-1

Heart Transplantation: Indications and Contraindications, Procedures and Complications
Catherine T. Fleming (Editor)
2010. ISBN 978-1-60876-591-1 (Online Book)

Heart Disease in Children
Marius D. Oliveira and William S. Copley (Editors)
2009. ISBN: 978-1-60741-504-6

Heart Disease in Children
Marius D. Oliveira and William S. Copley (Editors)
2009. ISBN: 978-1-61668-225-5 (Online Book)

Handbook of Cardiovascular Research
Jorgen Brataas and Viggo Nanstveit (Editors)
2009. ISBN: 978-1-60741-792-7

Comprehensive Models of Cardiovascular and Respiratory Systems: Their Mechanical Support and Interactions
Marek Darowsk and Gianfranco Ferrari (Editors)
2009. ISBN: 978-1-60876-212-5

Cardiac Rehabilitation
Jonathon T. Halliday (Editor)
2010. ISBN: 978-1-60741-918-1

Cardiovascular Signals in Diabetes Mellitus: A New Tool to Detect Autonomic Neuropathy
*Michal Javorka, Ingrid Tonhajzerova,
Zuzana Turianikova, Kamil Javorka,
Natasa Honzikova
and Mathias Baumert*
2010. ISBN: 978-1-60876-788-5

CARDIOLOGY RESEARCH AND CLINICAL DEVELOPMENTS SERIES:

CARDIOVASCULAR SIGNALS IN DIABETES MELLITUS: A NEW TOOL TO DETECT AUTONOMIC NEUROPATHY

MICHAL JAVORKA,
INGRID TONHAJZEROVA,
ZUZANA TURIANIKOVA,
KAMIL JAVORKA,
NATASA HONZIKOVA
AND
MATHIAS BAUMERT

Nova Biomedical Books
New York

Copyright © 2010 by Nova Science Publishers, Inc.

All rights reserved. No part of this book may be reproduced, stored in a retrieval system or transmitted in any form or by any means: electronic, electrostatic, magnetic, tape, mechanical photocopying, recording or otherwise without the written permission of the Publisher.

For permission to use material from this book please contact us:
Telephone 631-231-7269; Fax 631-231-8175
Web Site: http://www.novapublishers.com

NOTICE TO THE READER

The Publisher has taken reasonable care in the preparation of this book, but makes no expressed or implied warranty of any kind and assumes no responsibility for any errors or omissions. No liability is assumed for incidental or consequential damages in connection with or arising out of information contained in this book. The Publisher shall not be liable for any special, consequential, or exemplary damages resulting, in whole or in part, from the readers' use of, or reliance upon, this material. Any parts of this book based on government reports are so indicated and copyright is claimed for those parts to the extent applicable to compilations of such works.

Independent verification should be sought for any data, advice or recommendations contained in this book. In addition, no responsibility is assumed by the publisher for any injury and/or damage to persons or property arising from any methods, products, instructions, ideas or otherwise contained in this publication.

This publication is designed to provide accurate and authoritative information with regard to the subject matter covered herein. It is sold with the clear understanding that the Publisher is not engaged in rendering legal or any other professional services. If legal or any other expert assistance is required, the services of a competent person should be sought. FROM A DECLARATION OF PARTICIPANTS JOINTLY ADOPTED BY A COMMITTEE OF THE AMERICAN BAR ASSOCIATION AND A COMMITTEE OF PUBLISHERS.

LIBRARY OF CONGRESS CATALOGING-IN-PUBLICATION DATA

Cardiovascular signals in diabetes mellitus : a new tool to detect autonomic neuropathy / Michal Javorka ... [et al.].
   p. ; cm.
  Includes bibliographical references and index.
  ISBN 978-1-60876-788-5 (softcover)
  1. Diabetic neuropathies--Diagnosis. 2. Heart beat. 3. Blood pressure. 4. Autonomic nervous system--Diseases--Diagnosis. I. Javorka, Michal.
  [DNLM: 1. Diabetic Neuropathies--diagnosis. 2. Baroreflex. 3. Blood Pressure. 4. Diabetes Mellitus--physiopathology. 5. Heart Rate. WK 835 C2675 2009]
  RC422.D52C37 2009
  616.6'1075--dc22
                    2009048906

Published by Nova Science Publishers, Inc. ✦ New York

Contents

Preface		xi
Introduction		xiii
Section 1:	**Short-Term Heart Rate Complexity Analysis**	1
Chapter 1	Background	3
Chapter 2	Methods	5
Chapter 3	Results	13
Chapter 4	Interpretation	25
Section 2:	**Recurrences in Heart Rate Dynamics**	31
Chapter 5	Background	33
Chapter 6	Methods	35
Chapter 7	Results	39
Chapter 8	Interpretation	43
Section 3:	**Blood Pressure Oscillations – Linear and Multiscale Entropy Analysis**	45
Chapter 9	Background	47
Chapter 10	Methods	49

Chapter 11	Results	53
Chapter 12	Interpretation	57
Section 4:	**Linear and Nonlinear Analysis of Baroreflex**	**59**
Chapter 13	Background	61
Chapter 14	Methods	63
Chapter 15	Results	69
Chapter 16	Interpretation	75
Chapter 17	Conclusion	79
Acknowledgements		83
References		85
Index		95

PREFACE*

Early detection of subclinical autonomic dysfunction is of vital importance in patients with diabetes mellitus (DM) for the prevention of subsequent serious adverse consequences. Reduction in heart rate variability (HRV) is now regarded as the earliest indicator of cardiovascular dysregulation in DM. HRV has traditionally been quantified using linear (time and frequency domain) measures, which describe the magnitude of RR interval oscillations, but are insufficient to characterize complex heart rate dynamics. While HRV is mostly mediated by parasympathetic nervous system, beat-to-beat blood pressure recordings (blood pressure variability, BPV) may provide information regarding sympathetic activity. Assuming that heart and vessels are controlled by a nonlinear deterministic system, measures from nonlinear systems theory find increasingly more applications in cardiovascular signal analysis. A variety of novel measures has been developed to quantify nonlinear features of cardiovascular signals, providing information on the complexity of the dynamical system involved in the genesis of these short-term fluctuations. A loss of complexity is frequently observed in pathological states of the cardiovascular system suggesting that autonomic dysregulation represents a simplification of cardiovascular control since normal autonomic control results in complex system dynamics. Recent signal processing efforts aimed at quantifying the degree of synchronization between cardiovascular signals (e.g. cardio-respiratory coordination or cardiac baroreflex control). In our pilot study we demonstrated that novel nonlinear

---

* A version of this book was also published as a chapter in Handbook of Type 1 Diabetes Mellitus, edited by Leon Aucoin and Tritan Prideux published by Nova Science Publishers, Inc. It was submitted for appropriate modifications in an effort to encourage wider dissemination of research.

methods are often more sensitive to autonomic dysregulation than linear methods and therefore may improve the diagnostic power of cardiovascular variability analysis for cardiovascular autonomic neuropathy in DM. Our data indicate that cardiovascular dysregulation progresses in relatively short time frames, depending on the history of DM. Further, its progression appears to be associated with glycemic control. Different methods of cardiovascular variability analysis can provide mutually independent information and, therefore, should be used simultaneously for a comprehensive analysis of autonomic dysfunction to identify patients at risk for autonomic neuropathy.

INTRODUCTION

Diabetic autonomic neuropathy is one of the least recognized and understood complications of diabetes mellitus (DM) despite its significant negative impact on the survival and quality of life (Vinik and Erbas, 2001) due to its association with a variety of adverse sequela including fatal and nonfatal cardiovascular events (Liao et al., 2002; Whang and Bigger, 2003), ischemic cerebrovascular events (Toyry et al., 1996) and increased overall mortality (Wheeler et al., 2002).

Cardiovascular autonomic neuropathy (CAN) is the clinically most important form of diabetic autonomic neuropathy (Vinik et al., 2003). Early detection of subclinical autonomic dysfunction is therefore of vital importance for risk stratification in diabetic patients and an optimum management preventing serious adverse consequences (Schroeder et al., 2005).

Patients with DM who suffer from a parasympathetic dysfunction have usually resting heart rates that are higher than those of healthy subjects. In contrast, DM patients who suffer from a combined parasympathetic/sympathetic impairment might have heart rates lower than normal. Thus, heart rate itself is not a reliable diagnostic sign of CAN (Maser and Lenhard, 2005). Therefore, a simple tests battery (Ewing battery) was introduced over 20 years ago to diagnose CAN in a noninvasive manner. It includes several manoeuvres (deep breathing test, orthostatic test, Valsalva test, isometric handgrip test) during which heart rate and blood pressure changes are assessed. This battery has been widely adopted as a mean to classify CAN in terms of its severity, but it has a number of shortcomings as it (i) requires active patient participation and cooperation, (ii) is time consuming and (iii) is difficult to standardize. There is also a potential risk of adverse effects when the patient carries out these tests (Vinik et al., 2003; Takase et at., 2002). Alternatively, the analysis of spontaneous oscillations in heart rate during standardized conditions (supine rest, orthostasis) – heart rate variability analysis – has been proposed. It provides a rapid, sensitive, noninvasive and reproducible tool to assess cardiovascular autonomic dysfunction (Task Force of the European Society of Cardiology and the North American Society of Pacing and Electrophysiology, 1996; Makimattila et al., 2000; Burger et al., 2002).

Basic cardiovascular parameters, such as heart rate and blood pressure, continuously fluctuate over various time scales and are regulated by different control mechanisms with the aim to maintain homeostasis. The analysis of spontaneous heart rate and blood pressure oscillations (heart rate variability – HRV and blood pressure variability – BPV) therefore indirectly provides important information on the autonomic control of circulation under normal and diseased conditions as well (Parati et al., 2006; Baumert et al., 2009).

Reduction in HRV is now regarded to be the earliest indicator of cardiovascular dysregulation in DM. (Schroeder et al., 2005; Maser and Lenhard, 2005). Since HRV originates predominantly from oscillations in vagus nerve traffic (Eckberg, 2000), HRV analysis provides predominantly information on the vagal branch of the autonomic nervous system (Takalo et al., 1994). The reduction of spontaneous heart rate fluctuations found in diabetic patients with cardiac autonomic neuropathy therefore most likely reflects the advancing damage of the vagal nerve (Rollins et al., 1992; Ziegler, 1994).

The smooth muscles of the vessels and hence peripheral vascular resistance, on the other hand, are primarily under sympathetic nervous system control. The analysis of BPV might thus be useful for the detection of sympathetic dysfunction (Takalo et al., 1994; Cottin et al., 1999; Laitinen et al., 1999).

The human body is a complex adaptive system that enables a broad range of rapid responses required by continuously changing conditions, e.g. sleep vs. wake, rest vs. physical activity (Goldberger et al., 2002). Besides neural vagal and sympathetic pathways, cardiovascular regulation in the healthy human body is mediated by a variety of hormonal, genetic and external interactions. Output variables of that system (including heart rate and blood pressure), therefore, exhibit complex fluctuations on various time scales. Various disease states as well as aging appear to reduce this complexity, hereby reducing the adaptive capacity of the individual. Therefore, loss of complexity was proposed as a general feature of pathological dynamics (Baumert et al., 2004; Baumert et al., 2005; Costa et al., 2008; Voss et al., 2009).

In this book, we describe nonconventional data analysis techniques for HRV and BPV analyses and apply them to recordings of a group of young asymptomatic patients with type 1 DM. These methods are based on concepts from nonlinear dynamical systems theory and cover both, univariate (separate) analysis of HRV and BPV signals and bivariate time series analysis (i.e. analysis of synchronization between heart rate and blood pressure oscillations). The performance of nonlinear methods is compared to that of traditionally used linear analysis tools.

The book is organized into 4 major sections: 1) short-term heart rate complexity analysis; 2) recurrences in heart rate dynamics; 3) blood pressure oscillations – linear and multiscale entropy analysis; 4) linear and nonlinear analysis of the baroreflex. Each section begins with a short background followed by methods, results and interpretation.

Section 1: Short-Term Heart Rate Complexity Analysis

Chapter 1

BACKGROUND

HRV is traditionally quantified using linear measures in the time and frequency domain (Task Force of the European Society of Cardiology and the North American Society of Pacing and Electrophysiology, 1996) but these methods predominantly describe the magnitude of oscillations and are not sufficient to characterize the complex dynamics of heart beat modulation (Bettermann et al., 2001). In addition, although biosignal analysis by these methods usually detect the reduction of overall and beat-to-beat HRV in DM patients compared to a control group, there is a significant overlap in values of HRV measures between the groups (Javorka et al., 2005). Strong correlations between various time and frequency domain parameters and mean heart rate indicate that these parameters are not mutually independent and are not able to provide additional information useful for better discrimination of subjects with cardiovascular dysregulation (Colhoun et al., 2001; Liao et al., 2002). Therefore, the development of new parameters, which are able to quantify additional information embedded in the HRV signals is needed. Based on the assumption that the heart is controlled by a nonlinear deterministic system, measures from nonlinear systems theory are increasingly being used in HRV analysis. However, the application of traditionally used nonlinear methods (e.g. correlation dimension, largest Lyapunov exponent) is limited to long stationary signals – a condition that is only rarely met in physiology (Schreiber, 1999). We therefore employed measures that have been adopted to assess short-term HRV, ranging between epochs as short as 300 beats (Porta et al., 2001), 30 minute recordings (Voss et al., 1996), or up to a few thousands of heart beats (Costa et al., 2002). Although validity and reproducibility of those techniques have not been substantially investigated yet, studies based on 5 minute intervals suggest that they are better reproducible than frequency domain measures (Maestri et al., 2007; McNames and Aboy, 2006).

In this 1st section, we analysed HRV in a group of young diabetic patients by a set of nonlinear methods applicable to short (<1h) RR intervals time series. These methods enable to quantify different aspects of HRV not detectable by linear analyses – predominantly complexity. The major aim of this section was to test whether these new HRV measures provide diagnostic information regarding heart rate dysregulation and to assess their relations to standard linear HRV measures.

We hypothesized that heart rate regulation is significantly worsened after the follow-up period, indicating the progression of CAN. Therefore, the aim of this section was also to comprehensively assess short-term HRV in young DM patients before and after a 17 month follow-up, using set of standard time and frequency domain measures as well as novel nonlinear techniques.

Chapter 2

METHODS

SUBJECTS

We examined 17 patients with type 1 DM (10 women, 7 men) aged 12.9 – 31.5 years (mean ± SEM: 22.4 ± 1.0 years). The mean duration of disease was 12.4 ± 1.2 years. Based on anamnestic data, only one patient showed clinical symptoms of autonomic dysfunction (orthostatic intolerance). However, possible mechanisms responsible for the patient's orthostatic intolerance other than CAN could not be excluded. The Michigan Neuropathy Screening Instrument (MNSI), composed of a history questionnaire and physical assessment (foot sensation), did not reveal neuropathy in any patient, although one subject showed borderline values of suspected neuropathy. Physical examination (predominantly foot inspection) showed excessively dry skin in one subject. No other abnormalities were observed. In addition, vibration sensation was tested using a graduated tuning fork (128 Hz) applied to the dorsum of the patient's great toe. A reduced vibration sensation was found in one subject. Ankle reflexes were bilaterally present in all subjects. At the end of physical examination, standard monofilament sensation testing was performed at a pressure of 10 grams on ten separate places on both feet. All diabetic patients showed correct responses to these stimuli.

The patient group was compared to a control group consisting of 17 healthy gender and age matched subjects (mean age: 21.9 ± 0.9 years).

The study groups characteristics are given in Table 1. Seven subjects (4 in the control group, 3 in the DM group) were mild smokers with daily number of cigarettes less than five.

All subjects were instructed not to use substances which influence activities of the cardiovascular system (caffeine, alcohol) and refrain from smoking 12 hours before examination. All subjects gave their informed consent prior to examination. The study was approved by the ethics committee of Jessenius Faculty of Medicine, Comenius University.

Table 1. Study groups characteristics (control group – CON, group of patients with type 1 diabetes mellitus - DM). Values are presented as median (interquartile range) and *p*-values were obtained using Mann-Whitney U-test. Asterisk indicates significant (p < 0.05) between-groups difference

	CON	DM	p
Age (years)	22.1 (20.3-24.2)	23.3 (20.8-24.1)	0.617
Body Mass Index (kg m^{-2})	20.8 (19.5-23.6)	21.8 (21.4-24.6)	0.033*
Plasma glucose (mmol l^{-1})	4.9 (4.6-5.1)	8.6 (6.4-13.5)	0.001*
HbA_{1c} (%)	4.7 (4.5-5.0)	9.2 (8.6-9.9)	0.001*
Systolic blood pressure (mmHg)	124 (113-132)	117 (116-122)	0.326
Diastolic blood pressure (mmHg)	74 (64-76)	71 (68-77)	0.836
Duration of DM (years)	-	12.9 (10.4-14.2)	-
Age at DM diagnosis (years)	-	9.4 (8.2-11.6)	-

STUDY PROTOCOL

All subjects were examined over 60 minutes under standardized conditions in a quiet room from 8 to 12 AM. The subjects were instructed to lie comfortably in the supine position and not to speak or move unnecessarily. To ensure the subject's quiet state the data recording was supervised by an examiner and a nurse. The subjects were rested in the supine position for 20 min before the heart rate recordings started, allowing the cardiovascular system to reach equilibrium, i.e. a quasi-stationary condition. The patients and probands were asked to neither move nor speak during testing.

The VariaCardio TF4 device (Sima Media, Olomouc, Czech Republic) was used to continuously measure beat-to-beat heart rate (RR interval) recording at a sampling frequency of 1000 Hz, using a bipolar thoracic ECG lead. For HRV analysis we used the first 3200 beats of each recording (except for spectral analysis where the whole 60 minutes of recording were used). All ECG traces were visually scanned for artefacts.

DATA ANALYSIS

Standard (linear) HRV Analysis

Time domain analysis: for traditional time domain analysis of HRV we computed the three most commonly used measures as proposed by the HRV Task Force (Task Force of the European Society of Cardiology and the North American Society of Pacing and Electrophysiology, 1996):

- *meanNN* – the mean beat-to-beat interval of normal heart beats (NN denotes the normal RR interval);
- *sdNN* – the standard deviation of NN intervals – reflecting the overall magnitude of variability;
- *RMSSD* – the root-mean-square of successive beat-to-beat differences – reflecting the average magnitude of changes between two consecutive beats and regarded as a marker of vagal heart rate control.

Frequency domain analysis: For frequency domain analysis of HRV we analysed an epoch of 60 min. The RR interval time series was interpolated at 500 ms in order to obtain an equidistant time series, using cubic splines. As we were interested in oscillations between 0.04 and 0.5 Hz that are thought to be mediated by vagal and sympathetic efferents, we eliminated the slower oscillations and trends using the detrending procedure of Tarvainen et al. (2002). Subsequently, the power spectrum was repeatedly estimated, using fast Fourier transform (FFT) with the Hanning window length set to 1024 samples and a shift of 10 samples. The average power spectrum was computed and spectral powers obtained and the following measures were computed according to HRV Task Force recommendations:

- *LF* – low frequency power (0.04-0.15 Hz);
- *HF* – high frequency power (0.15-0.5 Hz);

Entropy Measures

In HRV analysis, entropy measures are used to quantify the complexity / regularity of heart rate fluctuations. Based on the framework of Shannon's information theory (Shannon, 1946), entropy is the measure of information of a given message, where a message with a low entropy /information is characterized by repetition. From the different techniques available to estimate information entropy we used multiscale entropy and compression entropy in this study.

Multiscale entropy (MSE): MSE was computed according to the procedure published by Costa et al. (2002, 2005). Given a one-dimensional discrete time series, $\{x_1,...,x_i,...,x_N\}$, we constructed consecutive coarse-grained time series $\{y^{(\tau)}\}$, determined by the scale factor τ, according to the equation:

$$y_j^{(\tau)} = 1/\tau \sum_{i=(j-1)\tau+1}^{j\tau} x_i$$

where τ represents the scale factor and $1 \leq j \leq N/\tau$. For scale 1, the coarse grained time series is simply the original time series. For higher scales, the coarse grained signal is constructed by the averaging of τ consecutive points without overlapping – this procedure reduces the length of each coarse-grained time series to N/τ. We calculated Sample Entropy (SampEn; Richman and Moorman, 2000) for each one of the coarse-grained time series plotted as a function of the scale factor.

SampEn is a refined version of traditionally used irregularity measure approximate entropy (ApEn; Pincus, 1995). It quantifies the irregularity and unpredictability of a time series. It reflects the conditional probability that two sequences of m consecutive data points which are similar to each other (within given tolerance r) will remain similar when one more consecutive point is included. (For details of the SampEn algorithm see Richman and Moorman, 2000). According to previous studies, we have chosen $m = 2$ and $r = 0.15$ * standard deviation of a time series. We have computed SampEn for scale values of τ up to 10 which corresponds to the minimal length of coarse-grained time series equal to 320 beats – the length acceptable for reliable estimate of SampEn (Richman and Moorman, 2000).

Compression entropy: A different way to assess entropy is based on data compression (Baumert et al., 2004). In information theory, the smallest algorithm that produces a string is at the same time the entropy of that string (Chaitin-Kolmogorov entropy; Li and Vitányi, 1997). Although it is theoretically impossible to develop such an algorithm, data compression techniques might provide a good approximation. We therefore applied a modified version of the LZ77 algorithm for lossless data compression introduced by Ziv and Lempel (1977) to compress the RR time series. To obtain inter values of RR intervals necessary for compression and to furthermore normalize the data to the HRV magnitude, all RR intervals were divided by 0.5 of its standard deviation and the numbers subsequently rounded. The ratio of the lengths of uncompressed to the compressed NN time series, is used as a HRV complexity measure and identified as compression entropy H_c.

Symbolic Dynamics

The concept of symbolic dynamics goes back to Hadammard (1898) and allows a simplified description of the dynamics of a system with a limited amount of symbols. For HRV analysis, the underlying theoretical concept is used in a rather pragmatic way. Here, consecutive RR intervals and their changes, respectively, are encoded, according to some transformation rules, into a few symbols of a certain alphabet. Subsequently, the dynamics of that symbol string is quantified, providing more global information regarding heart rate dynamics. We applied the two techniques based on Voss et al. (1996) and Porta et al. (2001):

According to the symbolic dynamics approach described by Voss et al, the series of RR intervals was transformed into an alphabet of 4 symbols {0, 1, 2, 3}. However in contrast to the original approach, we modified the transformation rule being based on the quartiles of RR interval distribution. Symbol '0' is given when the current RR interval lies within the 2nd and 3rd quartile (50th and 75th percentile) of the NN interval distribution, symbol '1' for above 3rd quartile (above 75th percentile), symbol '2' for RR interval between 1st and 2nd quartile (25th and 50th percentile) and symbol '3' for below 1st quartile (below 25th percentile). Thus, the dynamics encoded are not affected by the magnitude and shape of RR intervals distribution.

Subsequently, the symbol string is transformed into words (bins) of three successive symbols, e.g. '023' or '221'. The distribution of word types reflects some nonlinear properties of HRV. From this symbolic dynamics the following parameters were calculated:

- *FORBWORD* – the number of word types that very seldom occur, i.e. with a probability less than 0.001;
- *Shannon entropy* – Shannon entropy computed over all word types: a measure of word type distribution complexity;
- *Renyi entropy 0.25* – Renyi entropy with an a weighting coefficient of 0.25 computed over all word types, predominately assessing the words with low probability;

- *Renyi entropy 4* – Renyi entropy with a weighting coefficient of 4 computed over all word types, predominantly assessing words with high probabilities.

According to the symbolic dynamics approach described by Porta et al. (2001), the series of NN intervals was transformed into an alphabet of 6 symbols {0, 1, 2, 3, 4, 5}. As a transform rule, nonuniform quantization, keeping constant the number of points associated with each quantization level, was applied (Porta et al., 2007a)

Two approaches were used for analysis of the resulting symbolic time series:

- *Normalized complexity index (NCI)* was computed as a minimum of normalized corrected conditional entropy (NCCE) as a function of L (length of pattern). NCCE is a measure of the amount of information (corrected for short-term time series) carried by the L-th sample when the previous L-1 samples are known. NCCE remains constant in the case of white noise; decreases to zero in the case of fully predictable signals; exhibits a minimum if a repetitive pattern is embedded in the noise. NCI is a measure of the complexity of pattern distribution. It ranges from zero (maximum regularity) to one (maximum complexity). The larger the NCI, the more complex and less regular the time series.
- *Pattern classification*: all the patterns (symbolic sequences) with L = 3 were grouped into 4 families according to the number and types of variations from one symbol to the next (Porta et al, 2007b). The pattern families are: 1) patterns with no variation (0V, all three symbols are equal); 2) patterns with one variation (1V, two consecutive symbols are equal and the remaining one is different); 3) patterns with two like variations (2LV, the three symbols form an ascending or descending ramp), 4) patterns with two unlike variations (2UV, the three symbols form a peak or a valley). The rates of occurrence of these patterns are indicated as 0V%, 1V%, 2LV% and 2UV%.

Statistics

For statistical analysis we applied non-parametric statistics including median and interquartile ranges and the Mann-Whitney U-test for the comparison of group medians between controls and DM. Furthermore, we investigated the relationship between the different HRV measures using Spearman correlation coefficients. Results are presented as the median (interquartile range). A $p < 0.05$ was considered statistically significant.

Chapter 3

RESULTS

PATIENT CHARACTERISTICS

The diabetic patients had a slightly higher BMI compared to the control group, but all subjects were in the normal range (see Table 1). Patients with DM had significantly higher blood glucose and HbA$_{1c}$ levels. No between groups differences were found in blood pressure and all subjects were normotensive.

HEART RATE

The mean heart rate in the control group was 65.0 (63.0-70.4) bpm. In young patients with DM the mean heart rate was slightly but significantly increased (73.8 (66.4-79.3) bpm), as reflected by the decrease in meanNN (control group: 923 (852-952) ms, DM: 814 (757-904) ms; p = 0.048, see Figure 1).

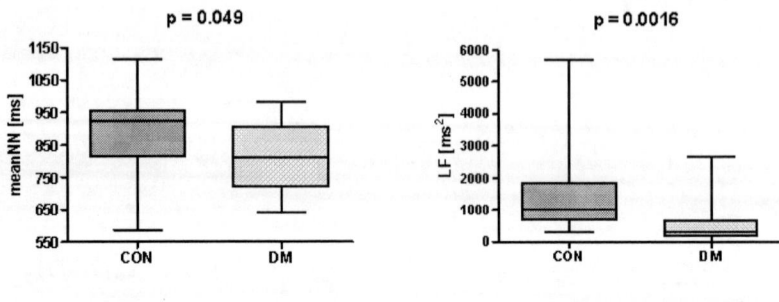
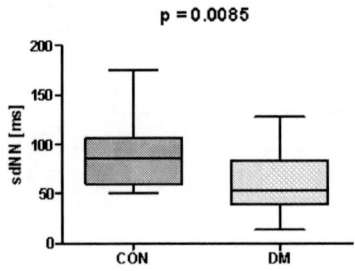
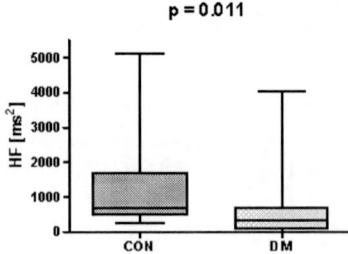
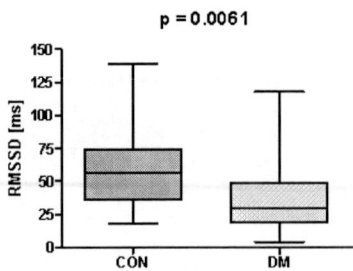

Figure 1. Standard linear time (left column) and frequency domain (right column) HRV measures all show a reduction in HRV magnitude in young patients with type 1 diabetes mellitus (DM) compared to healthy age and gender matched control group (CON) (Javorka et al., 2008a).

Traditional (Linear) HRV Measures

ime domain analysis of HRV, namely sdNN and RMSSD, showed a reduction in the overall HRV as well as in the magnitude of beat-to-beat differences in DM patients (Figure 1). After decomposing the heart rate time series into spectral components, the powers of both low and high frequency oscillations (LF, HF) were significantly reduced in DM patients, but varied considerably between individuals with large overlap between the two groups.

HRV Complexity Analysis

MSE

On scale 1, corresponding to the original time series without coarse graining, SampEn value was not statistically significantly different between the DM and control groups ($p = 0.125$).

On scales 2, 3, and 4, values of SampEn were found to be markedly reduced in DM patients ($p = 0.001$, 0.0002, 0.002 for scales 2, 3, and 4, respectively). In contrast, no significant differences in complexity were found on scales higher than 5 (Figure 2).

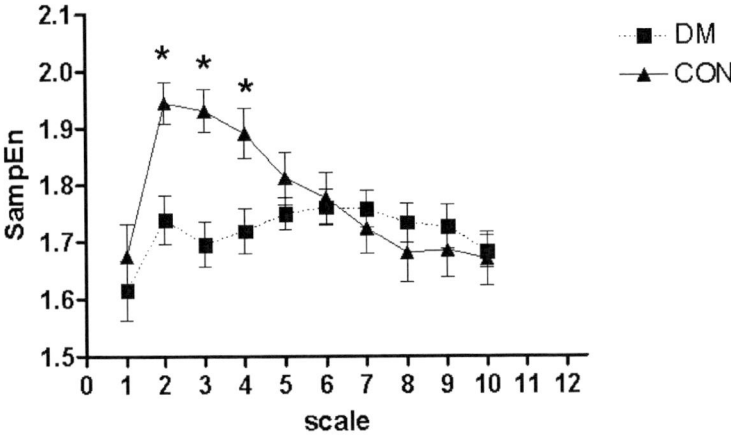

Figure 2. Multiscale entropy analysis of heart rate variability shows a significant reduction (asterisks) in complexity at small scales in young patients with type 1 diabetes mellitus (DM) compared to the control group (CON).

COMPRESSION ENTROPY

The compression entropy was significantly reduced in patients with DM (p = 0.0013, Figure 3).

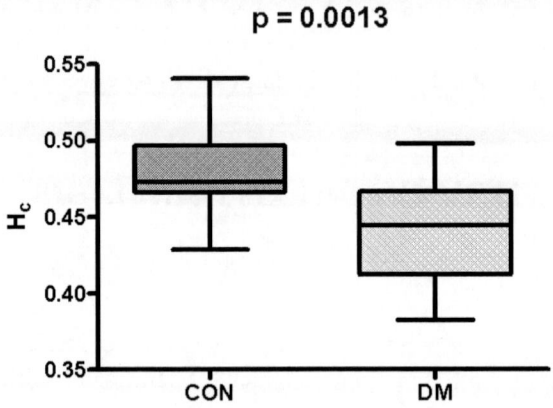

Figure 3. Compression entropy (H_c) of HRV in patients with type 1 diabetes mellitus (DM) and healthy controls (CON).

SYMBOLIC DYNAMICS

The entropy analysis based on symbolic dynamics by Voss et al. (Figure 4, left) revealed no change in complexity assessed by means of Shannon entropy, but a statistically significant reduction in the Renyi entropy was measured when a weighting coefficient of 4 was used (assessing word types with high probabilities). There was a trend for the number of forbidden words, (i.e. words with a low occurrence) to be higher in the DM group (p = 0.06), suggesting that the set of various patterns in HRV were less complex in DM compared to that in the control group.

From measures based on Porta's approach, we found lower normalized complexity index (NCI) in DM compared to the control group (Figure 5). Analysis of patterns consisting of three symbols revealed lower 2LV% in DM patients (Figure 4, right).

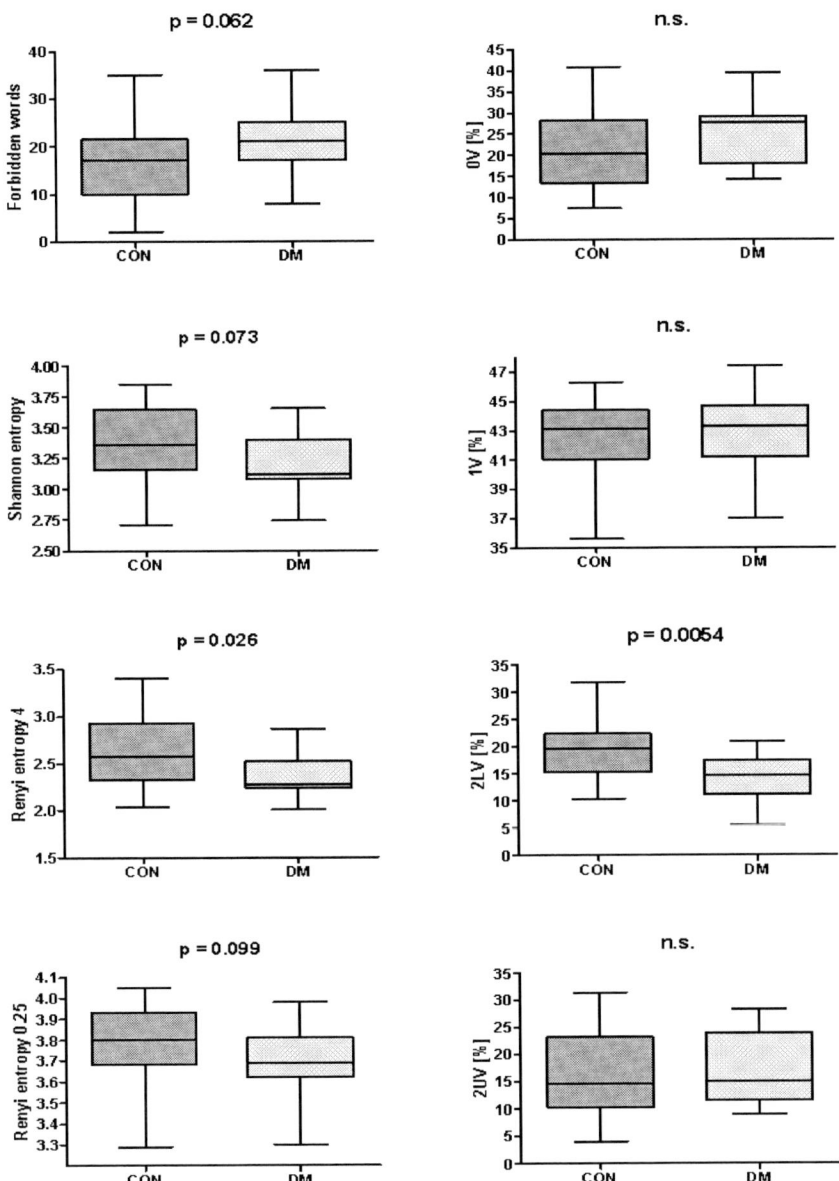

Figure 4. HRV measures based on symbolic dynamics according to the approach by Voss et al (left) and Porta et al (right) in patients with type 1 diabetes mellitus (DM) and healthy controls (CON).

CORRELATION ANALYSIS

Correlation analysis was performed between those HRV measures that were significantly different in DM patients when compared with the control group and thus are potentially useful for CAN assessment in DM.

All standard HRV measures were significantly positively correlated with each other in the control group as well as in the DM patients group. All HRV measures that were based on symbolic dynamics were found to be significantly correlated with at least one of the standard HRV measures in both groups, thus providing only limited additional diagnostic information. Similarly, the normalized complexity index (NCI) was significantly correlated with standard HRV indices.

Conversely, HRV measures based on MSE (scale three in controls and scales two, three and four in DM) showed no significant relationship with any of the standard HRV measures. The compression entropy H_c was not significantly correlated with standard HRV in the control group, but was in the DM group.

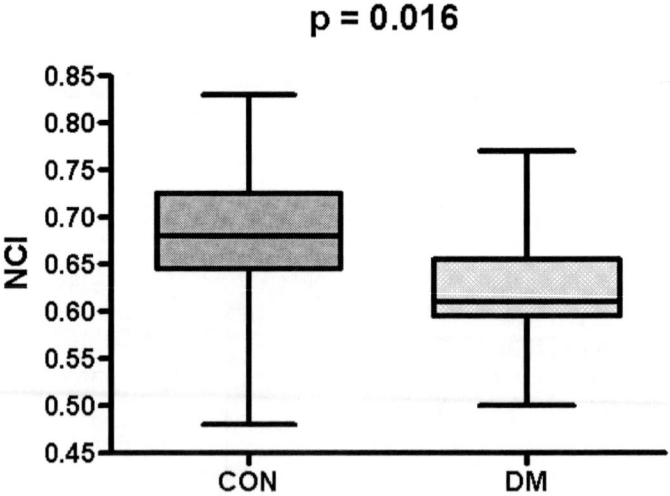

Figure 5. Normalized complexity index (NCI) of HRV in patients with type 1 diabetes mellitus (DM) and healthy controls (CON).

FOLLOW-UP ANALYSIS

We analysed a subset of 15 patients with type 1 DM (8 women, 7 men). Two patients from the original study were excluded as they were examined only once. The patients in this subgroup were followed-up after 16.8 ± 0.5 months (range: 15.0 – 20.5), using the same examination protocol. No changes in clinical MNSI measures were found.

Changes in HRV after the follow-up period of 17 months were assessed using the non-parametric Wilcoxon test for paired measurements. Further, we computed Spearman correlation coefficients (*rho*) between HRV measures and basic characteristics of diabetic patients during the 1st examination. To test whether changes in HRV are related to long-term glycemic control, we also computed correlation coefficients between the HbA$_{1c}$ values and differences in HRV parameters between the second and first examination (delta values).

Table 2. Characteristics of 15 diabetes mellitus patients during the inital investigation and after 17 month follow-up. Values are presented as median (interquartile range) and *p*-values were obtained using the Wilcoxon test for paired data. Asterisk indicates significant ($p < 0.05$) between-groups difference. BMI values were not available for the first measurement

	First measurement	Follow-up measurement	p
Age (years)	19.8 (19.4-22.7)	22.1 (20.3-24.2)	< 0.0001*
Body Mass Index (kg m^{-2})	-	21.6 (21.2-25.5)	-
Plasma glucose (mmol l^{-1})	10.5 (4.6-12.15)	8.6 (5.9-13.4)	0.79
HbA$_{1c}$ (%)	10.2 (9.1-10.7)	9.2 (8.7-9.8)	0.12
Systolic blood pressure (mmHg)	118 (112-130)	117 (116-122)	0.67
Diastolic blood pressure (mmHg)	80 (74-82)	71 (68-77)	0.02*
Duration of DM (years)	12.6 (9.4-14.3)	-	-
Age at DM diagnosis (years)	9.4 (8.2-11.6)	-	-

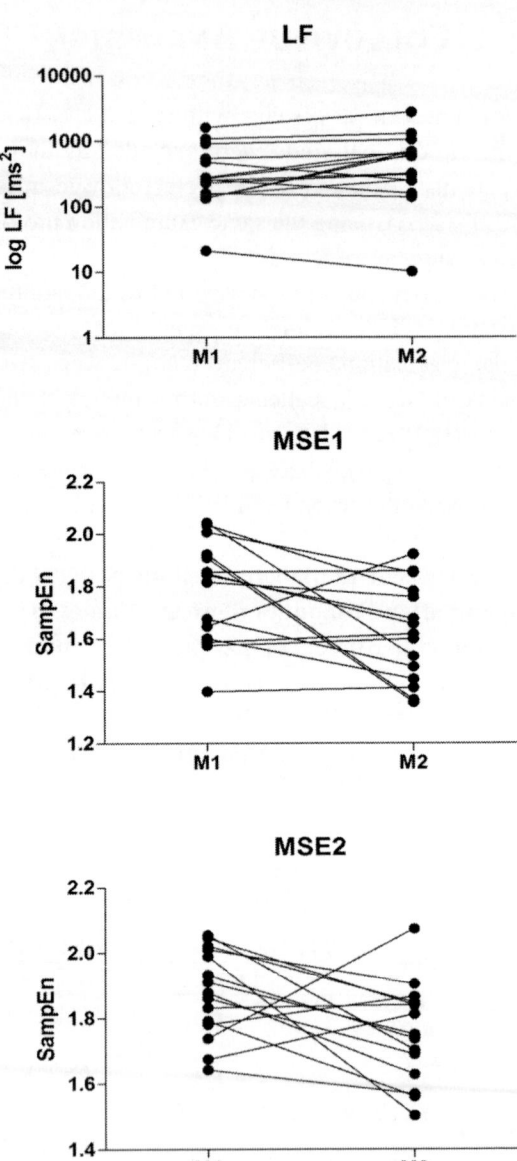

Figure 6. Individual changes in heart rate variability magnitude in low frequency band (LF) and in sample entropy values within multiscale entropy analysis for scales 1 and 2 (MSE1 and MSE2, respectively) before (M1) and after a 17 months follow-up period (M2). Significant increase in LF power and significant decrease in MSE1 and MSE2 were detected ($p < 0.05$, Wilcoxon test).

Clinical Characteristics After 17 Month Follow-Up

Basic characteristics of subset of diabetic patients included in the follow-up analysis are given in Table 2. Neither HbA_{1c} nor plasma glucose levels were significantly altered in our group of DM patients after a 17 months follow-up period. Diastolic blood pressure values were significantly lower during the 2nd examination.

Changes in HRV After 17 Month Follow-Up

HRV analysis by means of time and frequency domain measures revealed a significant increase in magnitude of low-frequency oscillations ($p = 0.02$; Figure 6, upper panel) of heart rate in DM patients during the follow-up measurement (Table 3).

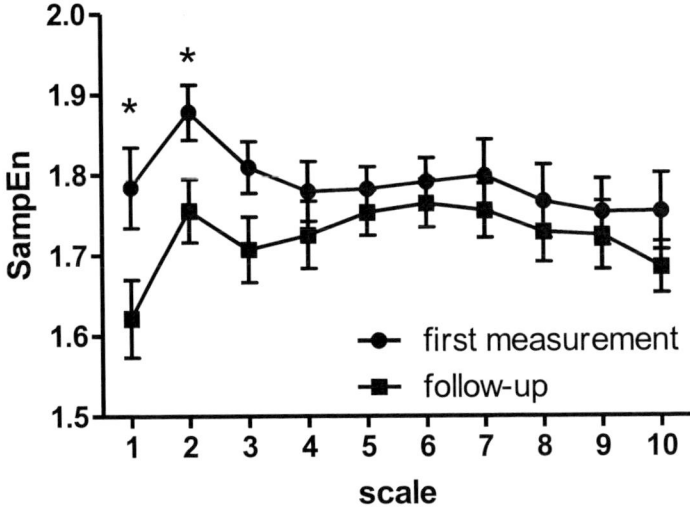

Figure 7. Multiscale entropy analysis of RR time series in 15 diabetes mellitus patients during the inital investigation and after 17 months follow-up. Values are presented as mean and error bars indicate SEM. Asterisks indicates significant ($p < 0.05$) differences, based on Wilcoxon test.

The complexity analysis of heart rate revealed a significant reduction in sample entropy values on scales one and two ($p = 0.03$; Figure 6, lower panels). The whole MSE analysis is illustrated in figure 7. None of the other complexity measures was significantly altered after the 17 month follow-up period.

Table 3. Heart rate variability measures in 15 patients with type 1 diabetes mellitus during the inital investigation and after 17 month follow-up. Values are presented as median and interquartile range (IQR) and *p*-values were obtained using Wilcoxon test for paired data. Asterisk indicates significant (p < 0.05) between-groups difference

	initial		follow up		
	Median	IQR	median	IQR	*p* value
MeanNN	766	684-836	814	766-905	0.21
SDNN	42	35-57	54	42-84	0.07
RMSSD	25	24-34	29	22-48	0.86
LF	259	155-509	575	248-674	0.02*
HF	265	214-483	328	131-695	0.78
NCI	0.69	0.62-0.73	0.61	0.60-0.65	0.23
0V%	18.9	16.8-23.1	27.5	19.6-28.3	0.11
1V%	42.2	40.8-44.1	43.9	42.0-44.7	0.22
2LV%	17.6	14.1-21.4	14.7	12.8-17.5	0.11
2UV%	21.2	13.6-23.7	15.1	11.8-22.5	0.36
Shannon entropy	3.45	3.21-3.56	3.12	3.10-3.36	0.28
Forbidden words	14	9-22	21	19-23	0.13
WPSUM02	0.22	0.20-0.27	0.29	0.25-0.29	0.16
WPSUM13	0.24	0.22-0.27	0.29	0.25-0.31	0.11
Renyi entropy 025	3.82	3.71-3.94	3.69	3.64-3.78	0.42
Renyi entropy 4	2.54	2.40-2.71	2.28	2.24-2.52	0.16
H_c	0.45	0.44-0.47	0.45	0.42-0.47	0.28

CORRELATIONS BETWEEN HRV AND CLINICAL DM PARAMETERS

The duration of DM was significantly correlated with HRV complexity as quantified by the symbolic dynamics measures 0V% (*rho* = 0.61, $p = 0.02$), 2LV% (*rho* = -0.74, $p = 0.001$), Shannon entropy (*rho* = -0.59, $p = 0.02$), WPSUM02 (*rho* = 0.54, $p = 0.02$), WPSUM13 (*rho* = -0.59, $p = 0.04$), and compression entropy H_c (*rho* = -0.59, *p* = 0.02). Neither time nor frequency domain HRV measures were correlated with the duration of DM.

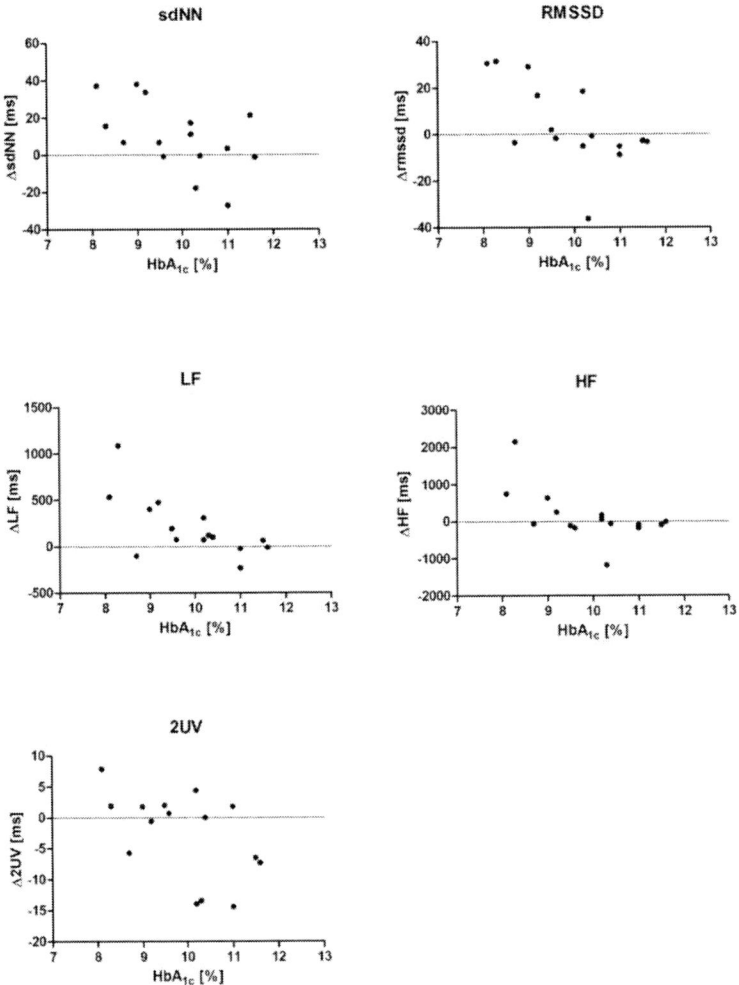

Figure 8. Scatterplots illustrating correlations between changes in heart rate variability (HRV) measures (delta values were obtained as the difference between values on the 2nd and 1st examination) and HbA$_{1c}$ values obtained during the 1st examination (for explanation of measures see Methods section). Each patient is represented by a dot. Patients with lower HbA$_{1c}$ values show an increase in HRV values during the follow-up measurement. Patients with worse long-term glycaemic control as expressed by higher HbA$_{1c}$ values show unchanged or decreased HRV values. All correlations were significant ($p < 0.05$).

None of the HRV measures was significantly correlated with HbA_{1c} or plasma glucose levels.

CORRELATIONS BETWEEN HbA_{1c} VALUES AND CHANGES IN HRV AFTER FOLLOW-UP

The change in HRV parameters sdNN, RMSSD, LF, HF and 2UV%, computed as the absolute difference between 2nd and 1st measurement, correlated negatively with the HbA_{1c} values (sdNN: $rho = -0.58$, $p = 0.02$; RMSSD: $rho = -0.65$, $p = 0.01$; LF: $rho = -0.66$, $p = 0.01$; HF: $rho = -0.57$, $p = 0.03$; 2UV%: $rho = -0.55$, $p = 0.03$). The correlations are illustrated by scatter plots (Figure 8).

Chapter 4

INTERPRETATION

The major finding of this first section was that the complexity of HRV was reduced in young patients with DM, pointing towards the pathological influence of diabetes mellitus on autonomic control. The complexity of HRV appears to be even more affected than the magnitude of HRV that is commonly assessed by cardiac autonomic neuropathy tests. Although most of the HRV complexity measures were significantly correlated with standard linear time and frequency domain measures thereby indicating vagal dysfunction, multiscale entropy and compression entropy seemed to provide additional diagnostic information on CAN in DM patients.

Beat-to-beat changes in heart rate are influenced by different regulatory processes, with a variety of hormonal, genetic and external interactions that act at different time scales resulting in complex patterns in the RR time series. Numerous studies have shown that quantifying complexity was of importance for the assessment of HRV (Batchinsky et al., 2007). This suggests that employing a multivariate approach based on a combination of linear and various nonlinear parameters will improve the diagnostic power of HRV. Reduced complexity in HRV is believed to result from a lower ability of regulatory subsystems to interact and was seen as a typical consequence of aging and disease (Porta et al., 2007a). Although CAN has been associated with heart rate dysregulation in severely complicated type 1 DM, the complexity of HRV has never been comprehensively studied in those patients.

STANDARD TIME AND FREQUENCY DOMAIN ANALYSIS OF HRV

Time domain HRV measures indicated a reduction in the magnitude of HRV in patients with DM, which has been previously described by other authors (Rollins et al., 1992, Javorka et al., 1999). Spectral decomposition of HRV into LF and HF power showed that this reduction was not linked to a specific frequency band. Since both LF and HF powers decrease with gradual vagal blockade (Martinmaeki et al., 2002), we conclude that impaired vagal heart rate modulation occurred in patients with DM.

ENTROPY ANALYSIS OF HRV

The most commonly used entropy measures are ApEn or SampEn, where the latter was an improved version of the former. Several authors observed reduced SampEn (or ApEn) in HRV after parasympathetic withdrawal upon standing, aging and mental stress (Javorka et al., 2002; Penttila et al., 2003; Vuksanovic and Gal, 2005; Batchinsky et al., 2007), implying that heart rate entropy was predominantly affected by parasympathetic nervous control (Hayano et al., 1991). Since ApEn and SampEn also return high values when they are applied to random data, they are strictly speaking not complexity measures, but regularity estimators. To overcome this particular limitation, Costa et al. (2002) proposed MSE measuring complexity in terms of a "meaningful structural richness". MSE enables the determination of information within relatively short signals on multiple time scales.

The comparison of ApEn between diabetics and controls was found not to be significantly different, despite a significant reduction in standard HRV measures in the diabetic group (Bettermann et al., 2001). These results are in line with our findings, which showed no group differences in MSE for scale one, which is equivalent to SampEn. Investigating larger scales according to the MSE procedure, we found marked reductions in SampEn ($p = 0.0002$) in DM patients for scales 2-4. These scales are thought to reflect mainly respiratory sinus arrhythmia supporting the concept of parasympathetic dysfunction in DM (Vinik et al., 2003; Javorka et al., 2005). In contrast, no significant differences were found on higher scales, implying that complexity was preserved for slower heart rate dynamics. The compression based entropy analysis also underpins the reduction in the complexity of short-term fluctuations of HRV found in our DM patients.

SYMBOLIC DYNAMICS

Symbolic dynamics approaches have been applied to HRV relatively frequently and it has been suggested that they provide additional prognostic/diagnostic information (Voss et al., 1998; Guzetti et al., 2005). When the dynamics of a quasi continuous signal are studied by means of a few symbols, appropriate coding is essential. We aimed to make our analysis independent of the magnitude and distribution of HRV using nonuniform symbol transformation as proposed by Porta et al. (2007a). The complexity analysis by means of the histogram of word types revealed a significant reduction in the Renyi entropy. Since the words assessed always consisted of three consecutive symbols they captured heart rate complexity within four heart beats, implying that vagal efferents predominately mediated these alterations.

The normalized complexity index (NCI) quantified complexity as the information carried by the most recent sample when the previous samples are known ("entropy rate"; Porta et al., 2007a) and was independent of the distribution ("static complexity"), only assessing the "dynamical complexity" as richness of a process dynamics. NCI has been shown to progressively decrease during the graded head-up tilt (Porta et al., 2007b) indicating that parasympathetic efferents are a major contributor. Our findings of reduced NCI in young diabetics could be also attributed to this change in cardiac control system balance.

Instead of assessing the complexity of words by means of the histogram, or the complexity index, the analysis proposed by Porta et al. (2007b) focuses on quantifying the contribution of basic patterns to beat-to-beat HRV. Only the measure 2LV%, representing the percentage of heart rate sequences monotonously increasing / decreasing, was significantly reduced in our DM patients. This indicates a reduced occurrence of sustained heart rate changes over three heart beats, probably a consequence of diminished respiratory sinus arrhythmia.

In summary our results obtained using various nonlinear techniques showed a reduced short-term complexity of HRV in DM that is predominantly under vagal influence (Beckers et al., 2006). Deriving information about sympathetic activity by means of HRV analyses appears to be rather difficult. Although a link between the LF rhythm of HRV and sympathetic activity has been found and the LF/HF (Furlan et al., 2000) ratio has been traditionally used as a surrogate marker of "sympathovagal balance", more recent studies have suggested that there are only little or no correlations between LF power and sympathetic outflow to the heart (Watson et al., 2007).

CORRELATION ANALYSIS

Correlation analysis showed that most of the complexity measures from various domains that have been investigated in this study are significantly correlated with linear HRV indices and might be of limited additional benefit for diagnosing CAN. In fact, the Mann-Whitney U-tests suggested that linear traditional HRV measures performed better in discriminating DM patients from controls. However, we identified two analysis techniques that may add significant information on CAN: multiscale entropy analysis and partly compression entropy. Both techniques show more pronounced differences between DM and controls in the Mann-Whitney U-test and furthermore no correlation with standard HRV measures.

FOLLOW-UP ANALYSIS

The magnitude of low frequency oscillations in heart rate was increased and the short-term complexity decreased in young patients with DM after a 17 month follow-up. In addition, HRV complexity measures were related to the duration of DM and moreover changes in HRV measures during follow-up period correlated with the long-term glycemic control.

The analysis of short-term heart rate complexity, utilizing a battery of modern non-linear techniques, showed a significant reduction in sample entropy after 17 month follow-up. This loss of entropy was only found after no (scale 1) or little coarse-graining (scale 2) of the RR interval time series, indicating that vagal efferents, that act fast predominately mediate these changes. Therefore, multiscale entropy analysis can be regarded a sensitive tool for the detection of subtle changes in heart rate control, even after a short follow-up period.

Autonomic dysregulation is thought to worsen with the progression of disease [9, 16, 19]. In our data of young patients with a history of DM ranging between 4 and 21 years, we found a significant relationship between loss of heart rate regulation and the duration of DM. It is important to note that those subtle changes in autonomic control could only be detected using nonlinear HRV complexity measures. The magnitude of HRV, as assessed by standard Task Force time and frequency domain measures, was not affected by the duration of DM.

In our study we found significant negative correlations between HbA_{1c} values and the change in all linear HRV magnitude measures and one of the nonlinear measures (2UV%) after follow-up. Interestingly, the patients with lower HbA_{1c} values showed even increase in HRV values during follow-up measurement. This unexpected increase could be attributed to seasonal effect and familiarization with examination protocol. No change or even decrease in HRV parameters was found in those patients that had higher HbA_{1c} values indicating worse long-term glycemic control.

Section 2: Recurrences in Heart Rate Dynamics

Chapter 5

BACKGROUND

Recurrence is a basic feature of many dynamical systems – it is defined as a repeated ocurrence of a given state of the system in time. Recurrence plot (RP) is a graphical representation of the recurrences in dynamical system (Marwan et al., 2007). The structures inside RP can be described quantitatively by the recurrence quantification analysis (RQA) (Webber and Zbilut, 1994; Marwan et al., 2002).

In this section we aimed to detect the heart rate dysregulation using RP analysis and to ascertain which of the RQA parameters are different in young patients with DM compared to control group.

BACKGROUND

Chapter 6

METHODS

SUBJECTS AND PROTOCOL

The same groups of subjects and protocol as in the 1st section of this chapter were used.

DATA ANALYSIS

The HRV analysis was performed off-line using special software on one time segment of RR interval time series - this segment consisted of 1000 normal RR intervals starting from 30th minute of supine rest.

First, a multidimensional state space has to be reconstructed from recorded time series that is one-dimensional. It can be performed by the method of time delay embedding (Takens, 1981). Each point in the reconstructed phase space represent the state of the system in a given time. This point is determined by m coordinates (embedding dimension). The values of these coordinates are the values from original time series delayed by selected time interval τ (time delay). Based on the modified false nearest neighbors method for computing of the minimum embedding dimension applicable on short time series (Cao, 1997) (we found saturation of E1 values for individual recordings in the embedding dimensions range of 7 to 10), and in accordance with previous studies (Dabire et al., 1998; Gonzalez et al., 2000;

Mestivier et al., 2001), we have chosen embedding dimension $m = 10$. Time delay (τ) for embedding was

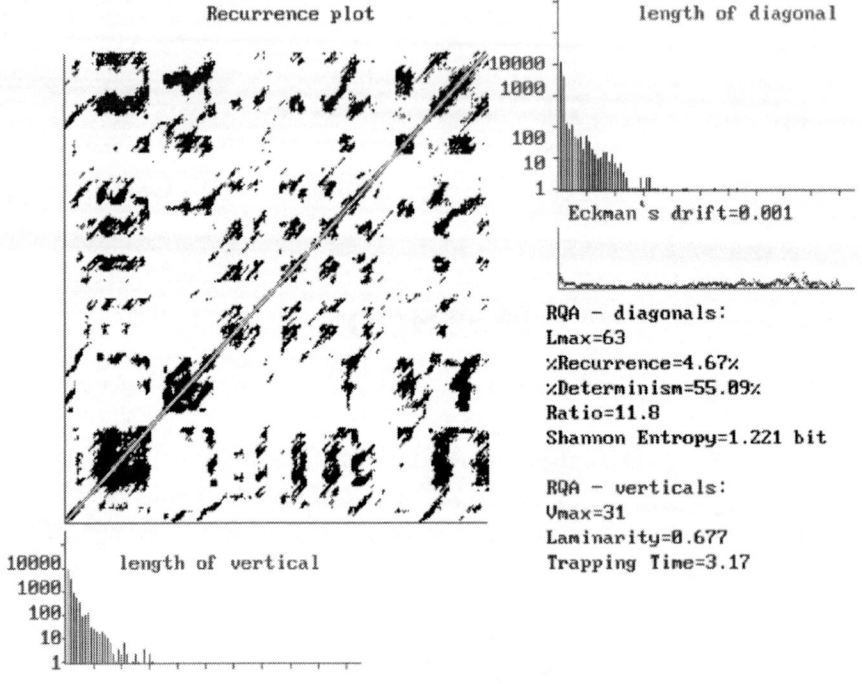

Figure 9. A representative example of the recurrence plot (RP) and the corresponding recurrence quantification analysis. Any recurrence of state in time i (x – axis) with state in time j (y – axis) is pictured on a matrix expressed by:
$\mathbf{R}_{i,j} = \Theta(\varepsilon - \|x_i - x_j\|)$, where $\Theta(.)$ is the Heaviside step function (if the number in parenthesis is higher than 0, the result will be 1; otherwise the result will be 0), $\|x_i - x_j\|$ denotes the Euclidean distance of two points in reconstructed phase space (x_i and x_j are the embedded vectors), and ε is an arbitrary threshold. Graphically, if the $\mathbf{R}_{i,j}$ equals to 1, black dot with the coordinates i and j occurs in the plot illustrating the closeness (within tolerance) of states in times i and j. In other words, the state in time i recurs later in time j (Javorka et al., 2008b).

set as the first minimum of the mutual information function (MIF) (Fraser and Swinney, 1986) individually for each recording to reduce relatively strong autocorrelation present in the heart rate signal. Next, the distances between individual points (a point in 10-dimensional space corresponds to a state of the system in given time) in times i and j were calculated using an Euclidean norm. When the distance of points was lower than given threshold (tolerance)

– a recurrence point in RP with coordinates [i, j] was plotted (Figure 9) (Webber and Zbilut, 1994; Marwan et al., 2007). The tolerance level was selected individually for each recording (for further details, see the last paragraph of this section).

The diagonals and verticals are the most important structures in RP. Diagonals reflect the repetitive occurrence of similar sequences of states in the system dynamics. The diagonals express the similarity of system behavior in two distinct time sequences. Verticals result from a persistence of one state during some time interval. These linear structures theoretically would not occur in random (stochastic) as opposed to deterministic process (Marwan et al., 2007).

Webber and Zbilut (1994) developed quantitative descriptors of the RP pattern – recurrence quantification analysis (RQA) measures. In our study, we analysed diagonal lines ocurrence using measure *%Det* (percentage of determinism) computed as the percentage of recurrence points forming diagonals from all recurrence points. Since the diagonals are a reflection of the repeating of states sequences, this parameter is a measure of the determinism and regularity of the system dynamics over time. The next parameter based on diagonal lines is *Lmax* - maximal length of a diagonal. We have also analysed parameters derived from vertical lines: Trapping time (*TT*) – mean length of the vertical lines, and Laminarity (*Lam*) - percentage of recurrence points forming verticals (Marwan et al., 2002). These measures were proposed as complexity measures. Simply said: the lower *TT* and *Lam* means the higher complexity of the system dynamics, because the state of the system stays for longer time in a state similar to previously occuring state.

For proper RQA measures evaluation, it is very important to properly set the tolerance level for recurrence points detection. The tolerance value should be selected so that percentage of recurrence points (*%Rec*) gives values between 0.1% and 2.0%. Larger tolerance values up to 5% may be necessary to obtain reliable values for *%Lam* and *TT* (Webber and Zbilut, 2005; Webber, 2007). Higher percentage of recurrence points in RP (higher *%Rec*) can itself cause higher probability of diagonals and verticals occurrence only by chance (in extreme situation, when *%Rec* = 100, all points in RP will form diagonals and verticals) and therefore almost all RQA parameters are usually dependent on *%Rec* value (the higher *%Rec* - the higher *%Det*, *Lmax*, *TT*, etc.). Therefore, to detect fine changes in structures of system dynamics recurrences, it is proper to construct RP with fixed *%Rec*. This procedure also minimize the influence of HRV magnitude on RQA parameters. We used individually chosen tolerance level giving the fixed *%Rec* = 5%.

Frequently, relatively strong autocorrelation is present in the heart rate signal – i.e. the length of two neighboring RR intervals is usually similar. As a consequence, the distance of two points in the phase space reconstructed from RR intervals, that are close in time, is usually small. Therefore, in recurrence plot, a lot of recurrence points in the vicinity of the main diagonal can be found purely as a consequence of above mentioned strong autocorrelation. To avoid the autocorrelation influence, Theiler window (Theiler, 1986) was applied and set to the value of time delay τ – i.e. only points more distant than τ from central diagonal ($j > i + \tau$) were considered for subsequent RQA measures computing.

STATISTICS

Given the gaussian distribution of parameters *%Det*, *Lmax* and *%Lam*, between groups comparisons were performed by two-sample t-test. Because of nongaussian distribution of variable *TT* and study groups characteristics, between groups comparisons were performed by nonparametric Mann-Whitney U-test for these variables. Values $p < 0.05$ were considered statistically significant.

Chapter 7

RESULTS

In Figure 9, an example of RQA analysis with corresponding recurrence plot is shown.

From RQA measures based on diagonal lines, we have found significantly higher percentage of points forming diagonals - *%Det* ($p = 0.038$, Figure 10) in DM. There was no significant difference in *Lmax* (Figure 11, $p = 0.760$) between these two groups.

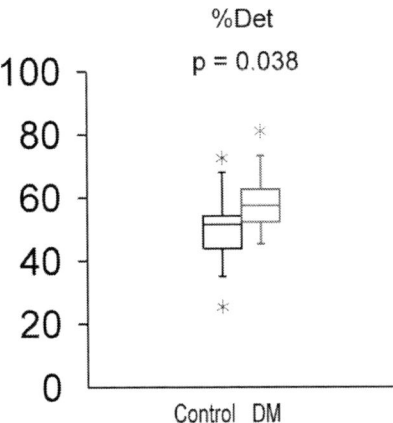

Figure 10. Box plot illustrating the comparison of percentage of determinism (*%Det*) between control group and diabetic group (DM). Box comprises interquartile range of values with central line corresponding to median. Asterisks correspond to outlier values.

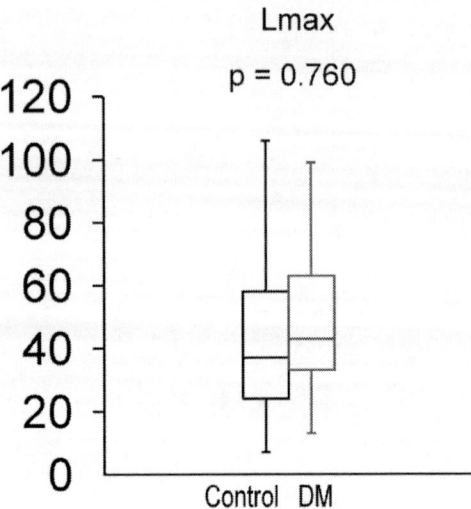

Figure 11. Box plot for comparison of maximum length of diagonal (*Lmax*) between control group and diabetic group (DM). Box comprises interquartile range of values with central line corresponding to median.

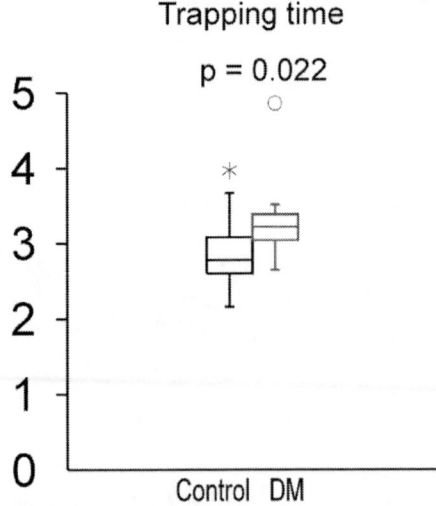

Figure 12. Box plot for comparison of trapping time between control group and diabetic group (DM). Box comprises interquartile range of values with central line corresponding to median. Asterisks and circles correspond to outlier values.

Using RQA measures derived from vertical lines, significant difference in *TT* was detected – *TT* was higher in DM subjects (Figure 12, $p = 0.022$). Other measure based on vertical lines - *Lam* (Figure 13) - was not significantly different between groups ($p = 0.084$).

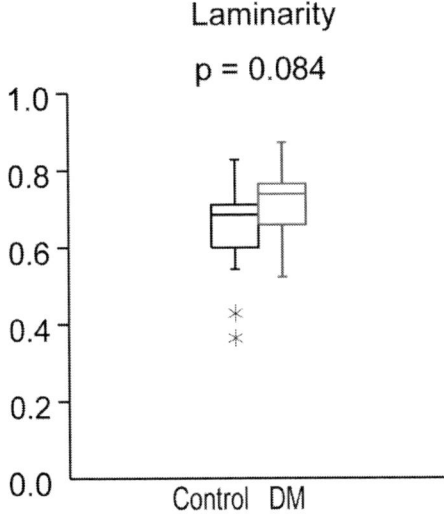

Figure 13. Box plot illustrating the comparison of laminarity between control group and diabetic group (DM). Box comprises interquartile range of values with central line corresponding to median. Asterisks correspond to outlier values.

Chapter 8

INTERPRETATION

The major findings of this section of our study are significant changes in measures derived from recurrence plot in diabetic patients. Higher percentage of points forming diagonals (*%Det*) and higher values of trapping time (*TT*) point towards complexity loss and simplification of heart rate dynamics in pathological conditions.

The major advantage of recurrence plots is their applicability to short and nonstationary physiological time series. The power of the recurrence quantification analysis also resides in its independence from constraining assumptions and limitations plaguing other analyses. Because recurrence structures are simply tallied within the signal, there is no need to pre-condition the data by filtering, linear detrending, or transforming the data to conform to any particular statistical distribution. For these reasons recurrence quantification analysis (RQA) has proven to be ideally suited for the study of numerous real-world systems (Marwan et al., 2007).

When applied to HRV time series, Dabire et al. (1998) and Gonzalez et al. (2000) observed significant increase of *%Det* and *Lmax* after parasympathetic blockade by atropine in rats. Similar resuls were obtained after administration of prazosine ($α_1$ - blockade) (Mestivier et al., 2001). These results suggest reduced complexity and better predictability of heart rate control after pharmacological simplification of the control system. Similar changes (higher *%Det* and lower *Lmax*) were found in an animal model of DM - in streptozotocin-induced diabetic rats (Giudice et al., 2002).

We used fixed *%Rec* = 5% in accordance with a suggestion of Webber (2007). Even after this adjustment, we have found an increase of *%Det* in young patients with DM, but parameter *Lmax* was not different in DM patients compared to control group. The difference between our results and results of above mentioned authors can be caused by using non-fixed *%Rec* in their studies. Nevertheless, our results point towards increased repeatability of heart rate patterns in diabetics suggesting reduced complexity of their heart control system (in accordance with results of Section 1 in this chapter). Similar RQA measures changes (although more prominent) were recently found during orthostatic test in healthy probands (Javorka et al., 2009).

RQA was traditionally focused on diagonal lines in recurrence plots, but additional information can be obtained from vertical lines characteristics. The vertical lines reflects the persistence of a given state of the system for some time interval (Marwan et al., 2007). In this study, we have shown that this phenomenon is more typical for DM patients compared to healthy control subjects. We suggest that this fact is the reflection of the reduction in heart rate complexity in diabetics. Loss of complexity has been proposed as a generic feature of pathologic dynamics (Goldberger et al., 2002). The results of our study (increased *%Det* and *TT*) are also in line with this concept of pathologically reduced heart rate complexity.

We suggest, that since heart rate is predominantly under parasympathetic nervous control (Hayano et al., 1991), the changes in heart rate dynamics recurrences are probably caused by parasympathetic dysfunction. Interestingly, none of analyzed RQA measures correlated significantly with the overall HRV magnitude as expressed by standard deviation of RR intervals (results not shown) in both groups. This finding suggests the importance of RQA parameters as the indices that are independent on the magnitude of HRV. These measures can provide novel information regarding heart rate dysregulation in DM patients.

Section 3: Blood Pressure Oscillations – Linear and Multiscale Entropy Analysis

Chapter 9

BACKGROUND

The reduction in heart rate variability (HRV) is well described in patients with diabetes mellitus (DM) and regarded an early sign of cardiac autonomic neuropathy (Ziegler, 1994). Contrary, the analysis of spontaneous beat-to-beat oscillations in blood pressure (BP) - blood pressure variability (BPV) - shows inconsistent changes with DM (Bernardi et al., 1997; Javorka et al., 2005).

Direct intraarterial measurement of blood pressure is the most precise method for its continuous monitoring. However, the usage of this method is markedly limited by its invasiveness (Porter et al., 1991). The volume-clamp method is the only alternative for noninvasive beat-to-beat blood pressure monitoring (Penaz, 1973; Virolainen, 1992). Although absolute values of the blood pressure obtained using this method can be distorted (overestimated systolic and underestimated diastolic blood pressures), volume-clamp method is able to reliably follow spontaneous blood pressure oscillations (Castiglioni et al., 1999).

Short term blood pressure changes are mediated mostly by sympathetic nevous system and therefore the analysis of short term BPV has been taken as more sensitive for detection of sympathetic dysregulation than HRV analysis (Takalo et al., 1994; Cottin et al., 1999; Laitinen et al., 1999). Only few papers were focused on assessment of short-term BPV in diabetic patients (Chau et al., 1994; Pecis et al., 2000; Watkins et al., 2000)

In the 1st section of this chapter we have shown that multiscale entropy (MSE) analysis was the most sensible method for detection of heart rate dysregulation in our group of diabetic patients. Therefore, in this part we focused on testing whether MSE analysis provides information about blood pressure dysregulation in young patients with DM according to the concept of complexity loss in pathological conditions.

Chapter 10

METHODS

SUBJECTS AND PROTOCOL

In this part we included a subset of 28 subjects from previous sections subdivided into 2 groups. The first group consisted of 14 patients with type 1 DM (7 women, 7 men) aged 22.3 ± 1.2 years (mean ± SEM). The mean duration of DM was 12.5 ± 1.4 years. We used the subset of a previously analysed diabetic group ($n = 17$) (see Section 1). Out of these 17 subjects, three were omitted because of artifacts (drift) in the beat-to-beat blood pressure signal.

The second group consisted of 14 healthy gender and age matched probands (mean age: 21.8 ± 1.1 years). All subjects gave their informed consent prior to examination. The same protocol as in the 1st section of this chapter was used.

Sixty-minute lasting recordings of RR intervals, systolic (SBP) and diastolic blood pressure (DBP) were obtained simultaneously and continuously under standardized conditions (supine position, rest, same time, same place) by means of a telemetric ECG system (VariaCardio TF4, Sima Media, Olomouc, Czech republic) and the beat-to-beat blood pressure monitor Finapres (Ohmeda 2300, USA).

DATA ANALYSIS

SBP and DBP oscillations analysis was performed off-line on a recorded segment consisting of 3200 beats using custom-made computer software. The analysis included linear (time domain) and complexity measures (multiscale entropy analysis).

Time Domain Parameters

BPV analysis. From SBP and DBP signals we computed the following linear measures:
For SBP: Mean SBP - mean systolic blood pressure value, SD SBP - standard deviation of systolic blood pressure values, RMSSD SBP - root-mean-square of successive differences of SBP values.
For DBP: Mean DBP - mean diastolic blood pressure value, SD DBP - standard deviation of diastolic blood pressure values, RMSSD DBP - root-mean-square of successive differences of DBP values.
SD SBP and SD DBP measures reflect the overall magnitude of BPV, whereas RMSSD SBP and RMSSD DBP quantify the beat-to-beat variability of the respective signals.

Multiscale Entropy (MSE)

MSE was computed according to the procedure presented in section 1. We have chosen a tolerance level of $r = 0.15$ * standard deviation of the time series to avoid distortion of SampEn values by changes in signal magnitude.

STATISTICS

Nonparametric tests were used to take into account the possibly non-gaussian distribution of BPV parameters. Between-groups comparisons (DM vs control group) were performed with the Mann-Whitney U-test. Discriminative power of the measures was assessed with linear discriminant analysis (step-wise backward variable selection; leaving-one-out cross-validation). Furthermore, we investigated the relationship between linear measures of HRV, SBPV and DBPV and SampEn values using Spearman correlation coefficients. A *p* value (two-tailed) < 0.05 was considered statistically significant. All values are presented as mean ± SEM.

Chapter 11

RESULTS

TIME DOMAIN PARAMETERS – BETWEEN GROUPS COMPARISON

Time domain BPV analysis. For both, SBPV and DBPV, no significant between group differences were found in the linear measures reflecting overall (SD SBP, SD DBP) and beat-to-beat (RMSSD SBP, RMSSD DBP) variability (Figure 14).

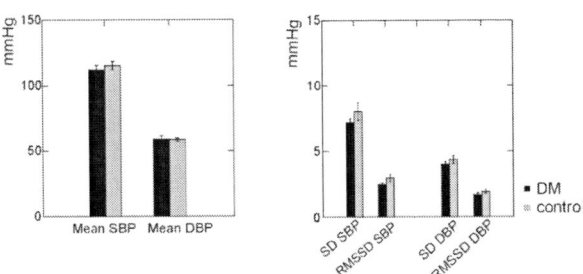

Figure 14. Linear time domain systolic blood pressure variability (SBPV) and diastolic blood pressure variability (DBPV) measures. No significant differences between controls and diabetic patients (DM) were found in the measures Mean SBP (systolic blood pressure) and Mean DBP (diastolic blood pressure), in the measures SD SBP, SD DBP (standard deviations of SBP and DBP, respectively) reflecting overall variability, nor in RMSSD SBP (root-mean-square of successive differences of SBP values), RMSSD DBP (root-mean-square of successive differences of DBP values), reflecting beat-to-beat variability.

MULTISCALE ENTROPY - BETWEEN GROUPS COMPARISON

MSE SBP analysis. Computing MSE from SBP signal, we observed a significantly reduced SampEn on scale 3 in DM patients compared to control group ($p = 0.039$). SampEn values on scales 2 and 4 were not significantly different in DM ($p = 0.077$ and $p = 0.066$, respectively). No differences were found on other scales (Figure 15, middle).

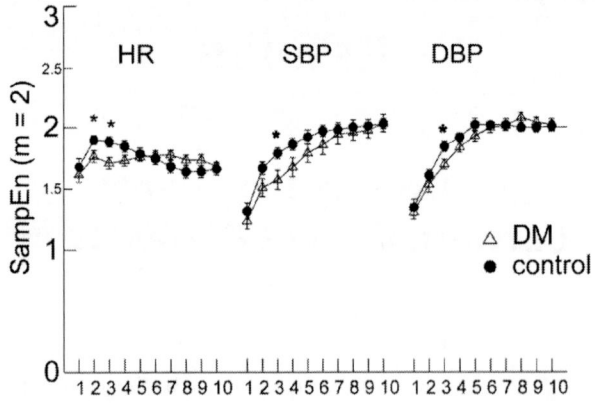

Figure 15. Multiscale entropy analysis (MSE). MSE shows a significant reduction (asterisks) in complexity at small scales (scales 2 and 3 for heart rate (HR) signals, scale 3 for both, systolic blood pressure (SBP) and diastolic blood pressure (DBP) signals) in young patients with type 1 diabetes mellitus (DM) compared to the control group (control) (Trunkvalterova et al., 2008).

MSE DBP analysis. Similar to the MSE SBP analysis results, the complexity was significantly reduced on scale 3 ($p = 0.015$) in patients with DM (Figure 15, right). (For comparison, also MSE analysis from heart rate – analysed in the 1st section – is presented in Figure 15).

CORRELATION ANALYSIS

Nonparametric correlation analysis was performed between time domain SBPV and DBPV measures and SampEn values of those scales that were significantly different between DM patients and control subjects.

SampEn values of SBP signals (scale 3) showed no signifficant correlation with overall (SD SBP) or beat-to-beat (RMSSD SBP) variability measures in the control group. In the DM group, SampEn values on that scale correlated positively with RMSSD SBP ($p = 0.006$) (Table 4).

Table 4. **Spearman correlation coefficients between systolic blood pressure variability (SBPV) measures and SampEn ($m = 2$) for the scale that was significantly altered in patients with diabetes mellitus (DM). The coefficients were separately computed for the healthy control group and for diabetic patients. MSE(3) denotes SampEn value for scale 3 within multiscale entropy (MSE) analysis. * - correlation significant at the 0.05**

Control group			
	Mean SBP	SD SBP	RMSSD SBP
MSE(3)	0.398	-0.007	0.248

DM			
	Mean SBP	SD SBP	RMSSD SBP
MSE(3)	0.526	0.189	0.690*

For DBP signals, SampEn values on scale 3 showed no significant correlation with standard time domain measures (Table 5).

LINEAR DISCRIMINANT ANALYSIS

Based on linear SBP and DBP measures, respectively, discriminant analysis resulted in a correct classification rate of 61% for each signal (selected variables: RMSSD SBP and RMSSD DBP, respectively). If MSE values were allowed to be selected the correct classification rate increased to 79% and 86%, respectively (selected variables for SBP: RMSSD SBP, SampEn at scales 4 and 7; for DBP: SampEn at scales 3 and 8).

Table 5. Spearman correlation coefficients between diastolic blood pressure variability (DBPV) measures and SampEn (m =2) for the scale that was significantly altered in patients with diabetes mellitus (DM). The coefficients were separately computed for the healthy control group and for diabetic patients. MSE(3) denotes SampEn value for scale 3 within multiscale entropy (MSE) analysis

Control group			
	Mean DBP	SD DBP	RMSSD DBP
MSE(3)	-0.064	0.176	0.506

DM			
	Mean DBP	SD DBP	RMSSD DBP
MSE(3)	-0.200	0.174	0.428

Chapter 12

INTERPRETATION

The major finding of this section is that multiscale entropy (MSE) analysis of BP signals allows a better discrimination between patients with type 1 diabetes mellitus and healthy subjects than linear time domain analysis. Further, MSE values are statistically independent from linear measures.

To our knowledge, this is the first study to investigate the complexity of beat-to-beat blood pressure fluctuations in patients with DM. No significant differences in SBPV or DBPV could be detected using linear time domain measures. Frequency domain analysis in the same group of patients showed nonsignificant changes of BPV (Javorka et al., 2005). This is in line with a previous study on BPV in DM (Chau et al., 1994). MSE analysis, however, revealed subtle abnormalities in both SBP and DBP dynamics in diabetic patients, emphasizing the high sensitivity of the MSE method compared to standard time domain techniques. MSE analysis might allow an earlier detection of sympathetic dysfunction in DM, which is thought to be mainly responsible for short-term blood pressure fluctuations (Laitinen et al., 1999). On the other hand indirect haemodynamic effects mediated by the heart might play a role.

For both heart rate (see section 1) and BP recordings, we obtained the best discrimination between patients and control subjects on MSE scale 3. In contrast, Costa et al. (2002) found the best discrimination between pathological (chronic heart failure) and healthy HR signals on scale 5. In addition, different MSE values were recently found for BP in patients with chronic heart failure compared to control subjects (Angelini et al., 2007) – the only application of the MSE method to BP signals so far. These results suggest that the scale optimal for discriminating pathological from physiological cardiovascular signals might vary with the type and stage of disease. Despite the analytical advantages of MSE its physiological meaning is not well understood. Furthermore, MSE analysis requires longer recording durations than conventional HRV/BPV analyses.

Section 4: Linear and Nonlinear Analysis of Baroreflex

Chapter 13

BACKGROUND

With beat-to-beat blood pressure measurement being available noninvasively via the volume-clamp method (Penaz et al., 1976), the neural modulation of the sinus node mediated by arterial baroreceptors has become quantifyable (baroreflex sensitivity; BRS) (Ziegler et al. 1992; Vinik and Ziegler 2007).

Decreased BRS was found in both type 1 and type 2 DM patients, using time domain (sequence method) and frequency domain (cross-spectral method) analyses (Frattola et al., 1997; Ruiz et al., 2005; Boysen et al., 2007). Compared to HRV analysis, BRS measures were found in several studies to have a higher sensitivity to detect the cardiovascular dysregulation in DM (Frattola et al., 1997; Bernardi, 2000; Loimaala et al,. 2003).

Both, experimental studies and mathematical models on the cardiovascular control system (Cavalcanti and Belardinelli, 1996; Cerutti et al., 2006; Raab et al. 2006) indicate that significant nonlinear components are involved. In previous sections of this chapter, we showed that nonlinear HRV analysis methods are more sensitive to cardiovascular dysregulation in type 1 DM patients than linear measures. Based on these findings we hypothesized that recently developed nonlinear methods for the quantification of synchronization between signals (e.g. blood pressure and heart rate) are more sensitive to baroreflex impairment in young patients with type 1 DM than standard BRS indices.

The aim of this section was therefore to employ those novel nonlinear synchronization approaches to heart rate and blood pressure data and to compare their performance to various linear standard BRS methods.

Chapter 14

METHODS

SUBJECTS AND PROTOCOL

The same groups of subjects and protocol as in the 3rd section of this chapter were used.

Sixty-minute lasting beat-to-beat recordings of systolic blood pressure (SBP) and pulse intervals (PI) were obtained continuously under standardized conditions (supine position, rest, same time, same place) by means of the beat-to-beat blood pressure monitor Finapres (Ohmeda 2300, USA). PI was defined as the time interval between two successive blood pressure peaks corresponding to SBP values.

DATA ANALYSIS

Analysis was performed off-line on a recording segment consisting of 3200 beats using custom-made computer software. The analysis included quantification of various baroreflex sensitivity measures and nonlinear synchronization.

Baroreflex Sensitivity Measurement

All BRS indices were computed from the whole 60 min of recordings of SBP and PI.

Sequence Method

SBP time series are scanned for sequences of monotonously increasing / decreasing blood pressure values over at least 3 consecutive heart beats that are parralled by sequences of monotonously increasing / decreasing values in PI shifted by one heart beat (Mancia et al., 1986). Such sequences are interpreted as cardiac baroreflex response to blood pressure increases / decreases. If the correlation coefficient computed between the SPB and PI sequences is > 0.8 the sequence is considered valid and linear regression slope is computed for that ‚baroreflex' sequence. We computed average slopes for bradycardic (an increase in blood pressure accompanied by an increase in PI) and tachycardic (a decrease in blood pressure accompanied by a decrease in PI) sequences (*bslope* and *tslope* indices, respectively).

Time Domain Cross-Correlation Method

The time domain cross-correlation technique was used for calculation of BRS value and time delay between SBP and PI signals (Westerhof et al., 2004). Beat-to-beat values of PI and SBP are interpolated at 1-s intervals using cubic splines. Subsequently, cross-correlation coefficients between 10-s series of PI and SBP are computed for delays in PI of 0-10 s. Mean value of the time delay of all 10-s sequences that gives the highest correlation between both signals was computed – *xBRS delay*. In addition, we computed the mean slope of all 10-s sequences – *xBRS* value.

Cross-Spectral Method

BRS was assessed by the cross-spectral method (Zavodna et al., 2006). Equidistant time series of SBP and PI were obtained by linear interpolation between the neighbouring values at a sampling interval of 250 ms. Linear trends were then removed by the least-squares approximation method. The autocorrelation of the SBP sequence and the cross-correlation functions between SBP and PI sequences were calculated next. The power spectrum of SBP time sequence was calculated as the spectrum of autocorrelation of SBP sequence, and the cross-spectrum between SBP and PI sequences was calculated from the cross-correlation function between SBP and PI intervals. A Hanning window was used for the Gipson effect removal. The coherence factor and the transfer function gain as a quotient between the cross-spectrum of SBP and PI intervals and the power spectrum of SBP were calculated.

The values of baroreflex sensitivity (*BRS index*) were determined in the frequency range from 0.04 to 0.15 Hz of the transfer function, at the highest coherence. This value was taken into account only if the coherence was higher than 0.5. In case that more than one peak was present in this range, the sum of values of coherence was taken as 1 and the corresponding BRS value was taken into account with respect to the weight of the actual coherence in a summed coherence value. The *BRSf index* was calculated by the identical technique but instead of PI, beat-to-beat instantaneous values of heart rate were used.

Analysis of Nonlinear Synchronization

Since nonlinear synchronization indices are influenced by the number of beats used for their calculation, we have computed following indices for the 1st-3200th beats of recordings.

Information Domain Synchronization Index (IDSI)

The information domain synchronization index (*IDSI*) quantifies the maximum amount of information exchange between PI and SBP signals and was calculated according the algorithm described by Porta et al. (1999, 2000). It quantifies the amount of information that is carried over to the present sample of a signal based on the known pattern of L-1 previous samples of a second signal (the pattern length L is varied to obtain optimal predictability). Thus, this index quantifies to what extent a signal can be predicted from another signal – when SBP and PI signals are uncoupled IDSI is equal to 0, while it equals 1 in the case of complete synchronization.

The first step of an algorithm for IDSI computation is to encode SBP and PI time series into set of limited number of symbols. We have used two encoding rules: regular encoding (6 symbols, equal width of the range of values used for each symbol) – *IDSIreg*, and equiprobable encoding (6 symbols, each symbol occuring with equal frequency) – *IDSIeq*.

Cross Multiscale Entropy (CrossMSE)

Cross Sample Entropy (*Cross-SampEn*) was recently introduced as an index of asynchrony and dissimilarity between two signals, where lower values correspond to a higher degree of the signals' joint synchrony (Richman and Moorman, 2000). The index was computed on normalized time series, obtained by subtracting the signal mean values and subsequent division by the time series' standard deviations.

Since cardiovascular parameters oscillate on various time scales we extended the originally proposed method by computing *Cross-SampEn* values for various time scales using coarse-grained signals according to concept of Costa et al. (2002). For both, PI and SBP signals, coarse-grained time series for scale τ were obtained by taking the arithmetic mean of the τ neighbouring original values without overlapping. For scale 1, the coarse grained time series are simply the original time series. We calculated *Cross-SampEn* for each coarse-grained time series pairs and plotted the results as a function of the scale factor - the resulting curve describes the Cross-Multiscale Entropy Analysis (*Cross-MSE*).

Cross-MSE was computed for various combinations of input parameters m ($m = 1$ and 2) and r ($r = 0.15$ and 0.3).

Joint Symbolic Dynamics

Changes between consecutive PI and SBP intervals, respectively, are transformed into symbol sequences consisting of ‚0' and ‚1' encoding a decrease and increase between consecutive PI/SBP values, respectively (Baumert et al., 2002; Baumert et al., 2005). Subsequently, the probability of word types consisiting of 3 consecutive PI and SBP symbols is analyzed. Given the two different symbol types and a word length of 3, there are $2^3 * 2^3 = 64$ different word types. From these 64 different word types we focus our analysis on the portions of symmetric word types (*JSDsym*) where the pattern in SBP is equal to the pattern in PI, reflecting baroreflex-like response patterns and diametric word types (*JSDdiam*), where the PI response to SBP changes is assymetric and opposite to that of baroreflex.

Information-Based Similarity Index

Similar to the previous method, the first step of computing the information-based similarity index – *IBSI* – involves symbolization (Yang et al., 2003). Changes in successive values of PI and SBP, respectively, were encoded as ‚1' if an increase and as ‚0' if a decrease in respective time series occured. We considered words of k-bit length, shifting one data point at a time. Thus, the algorithm produces a collection of k-bit words over the whole time series. For analysis of dynamics similarity encompassing various number of heart beats, we varied length of word (k) from 3 to 10. We counted the occurrences of different word types, and subsequently sorted them in descending order by frequency of occurrence. The resulting rank-frequency distribution represents the statistical hierarchy of symbolic words. Therefore, the first rank word corresponds to the type of fluctuation which is the most frequent pattern in the time series.

In the next step, the rank order difference between PI and SBP time series was visualized by plotting the rank number of each k-bit word in the first time series against that of the second time series. The distance (or dissimilarity) between PI and SBP time series was quantified by measuring the scatter of these points. If two time series are similar in their rank order of the words, the scattered points will be located near the diagonal line. Therefore, the average deviation of these scattered points away from the diagonal line is a measure of the "distance" between these two time series. The resulting distance is expressed as an IBSI value from interval [0; 1] - greater distance indicates less similarity and vice versa.

STATISTICS

Nonparametric tests were used to take into account the non-gaussian distribution of the analyzed parameters. Between-groups comparisons (DM vs control group) were performed with the Mann-Whitney U-test. To assess relations between various measures, we computed Spearman correlation coefficients. A p value (two-tailed) < 0.05 was considered statistically significant.

Chapter 15

RESULTS

BAROREFLEX SENSITIVITY – BETWEEN GROUPS COMPARISON

The sequence method revealed a significant decrease in the slope of bradycardic baroreflex responses (lower *bslope*, $p = 0.035$) in the DM group while only tendency towards the reduction of tachycardic responses slope (*tslope*, $p = 0.141$) was observed (Figure 16).

While the *xBRS* index based on the cross-correlation method did not reveal a significant difference between both groups, we observed a significant increase in baroreflex loop time delay (*xBRS delay*, $p = 0.007$) in young patients with DM compared to the control group (Figure 17).

None of the cross-spectral method measures (*BRS* and *BRSf indices*, $p = 0.098$ and 0.198, respectively) was significantly different between groups (Figure 18). However, a marginally nonsignificant reduction ($p = 0.054$) in coherence values between systolic blood pressure and PI signal was found.

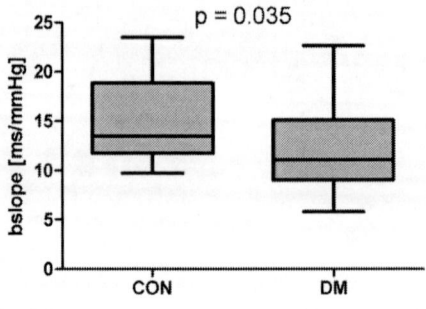

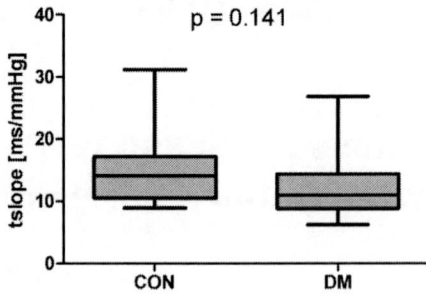

Figure 16. Baroreflex sensitivity assessed by sequence method was calculated separately for bradycardic (*bslope*) and tachycardic (*tslope*) sequences. Significantly reduced bslope was found in patients with diabetes mellitus (DM) compared to control group (CON). No significant difference in *tslope* parameter was found. Box plots illustrate medians and interquartile ranges.

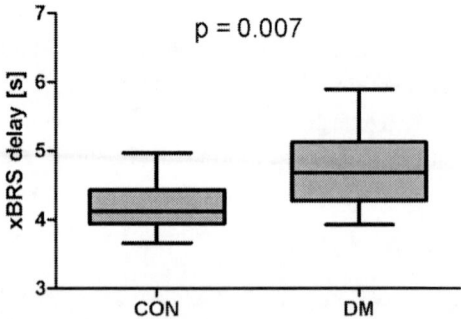

Figure 17. Difference in time delay within baroreflex loop (*xBRS delay*) between control group (CON) and patients with diabetes mellitus (DM) assessed by time domain cross-correlation method.

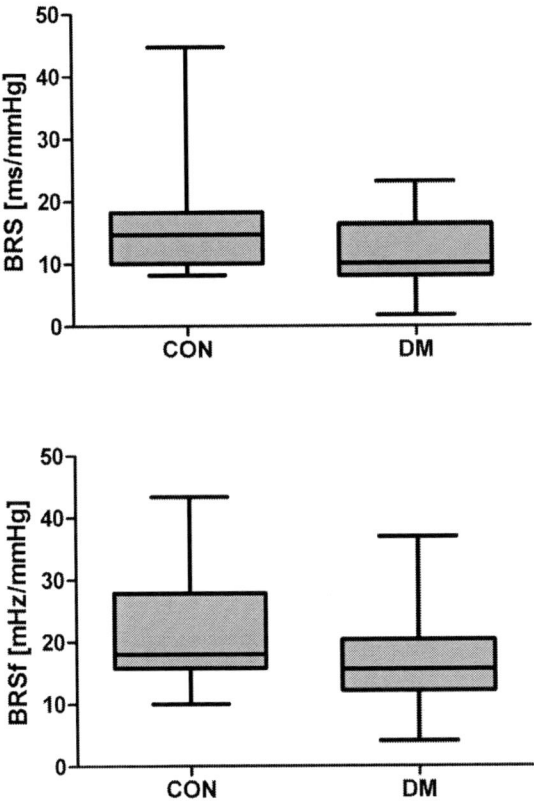

Figure 18. Baroreflex sensitivity calculated with the cross-spectral method from pulse interval vs. systolic blood pressure (*BRS*) and from heart rate vs. systolic blood pressure (*BRSf*). Although both indices showed a tendency towards lower values in patients with diabetes mellitus (DM) compared to control subjects (CON), no significant differences were found. Box plots illustrate medians and interquartile ranges.

NONLINEAR SYNCHRONIZATION – BETWEEN GROUPS COMPARISON

No significant between groups differences were found neither in *IDSIreg* nor in *IDSIeq* ($p = 0.908$ and 0.421, respectively). Similarly, CrossMSE analysis (using various combinations of m (for $m = 1$ and 2) and r (for $r = 0.15$ and 0.30) parameters) was not able to detect a significant difference in SBP/PI synchronization between the DM and control groups (*p* values ranged from 0.141 to 0.982 for scales 1-10) (Figure 19). Measures based on JSD method were also not able to detect any difference between both groups (for *JSDsym* and *JSDdiam*: $p = 0.818$ and 0.358, respectively).

In contrast, Yang`s IBSI tended to be higher (indicating lower similarity/synchronization of SBP and PI signals) in diabetics compared to control group for all assessed lengths of word (*k* ranging from 3 to 10). For word length of 4, a statistically significant increase in IBSI was found in the DM group ($p = 0.039$, Figure 20).

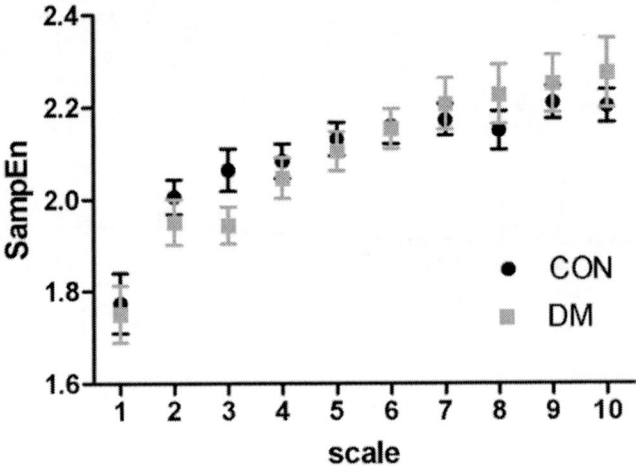

Figure 19. Cross multiscale entropy analysis (Cross-MSE) for scales 1-10. No statistically significant differences between control subjects (CON) and patients with type 1 diabetes mellitus (DM) were found. The presented results were obtained using $m = 2$ and $r = 0.15$. Similar results were obtained with other combinations of the parameters *m* and *r*. Values are presented as mean and SEM.

CORRELATIONS BETWEEN SIGNIFICANTLY ALTERED MEASURES

There were no significant correlations among *IBSI*, *xBRS delay*, *bslope* in the control group. Contrary, *xBRS delay* was negatively correlated with bslope ($r = -0.69$, $p = 0.006$) in the DM group (Table 6).

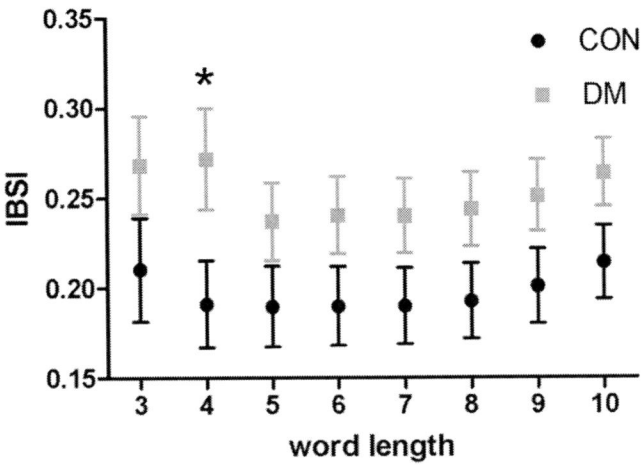

Figure 20. Information based similarity indices (*IBSI*) for various word lengths. *IBSI* values showed a consistent tendency to be higher for all word lengths in young diabetic patients (DM). The difference was statistically significant for word length of 4 ($p = 0.039$). Values are presented as mean and SEM.

Table 6. Spearman correlation coefficients among significantly altered baroreflex / PI/SBP synchronization measures in the control group (top) and in patients with diabetes mellitus (bottom). IBSI4 denotes the information-based similarity index with the length of words equal to 4.

	IBSI4	bslope
bslope	0.13	
xBRS delay	0.35	-0.43

	IBSI4	bslope
bslope	-0.32	
xBRS delay	0.47	-0.69*

Chapter 16

INTERPRETATION

The major finding of this section is the relatively well-preserved baroreflex sensitivity in young patients with type 1 diabetes mellitus that is accompanied by an increased time delay within the baroreflex loop and a decrease in the level of synchronization between blood pressure and heart rate fluctuations.

Unlike HRV analysis, the suitability of BRS assessment to diagnose autonomic neuropathy in DM is not well-established. Although reduced baroreflex sensitivity (BRS) has been repeatedly proposed to be an early sign of autonomic dysfuncion in DM patients (e.g. (Frattola et al., 1997; Ziegler et al., 1992)), several studies reported preserved baroreflex function (Ducher et al., 2001; Sanya et al., 2003) in DM. In our group of young diabetic patients, baroreflex sensitivity as assessed by various methods was relatively well-preserved. In previous sections, we reported impaired heart rate control, most significantly expressed by lower complexity values of HRV. This would suggest that, in the time course of diabetic autonomic impairment, reduced HRV can be detected earlier than baroreflex dysregulation. This is in line with the observation that vagal nerve damage, predominantly mediating HRV, precedes sympathetic nerve damage, mediating autonomic vascular responses.

COMPARISON OF ESTABLISHED BRS TECHNIQUES

The baroreflex assessment techniques applied in this study quantify partly different features of heart rate and blood pressure time series and therefore perform slightly different.

One of the sequence method's advantages over other employed techniques is its ability to quantify the slopes of PI responses to increase and decrease of blood pressure separately. Interestingly, we found reduced slope of bradycardic baroreflex sequences while the slope of tachycardic sequences was preserved in DM groups. Such asymmetric impairment was previously observed with pharmacological baroreflex assessment (Oxford method) in diabetic humans (Eckberg et al., 1986) and rats (Ducher et al., 1999).

The relatively lower sensitivity of cross-spectral and cross-correlation methods to detect changes in baroreflex sensitivity in our group of diabetics might therefore be attributed to their inability to analyse separately brady/tachycardic baroreflex events.

Previous baroreflex studies have shown that not only static property (gain), but also the dynamic property (time delay) of the reflex loop determines its efficiency (Gulli et al., 2003). The baroreflex time delay is elevated in healthy subjects during orthostatic challenge (Westerhof et al., 2004) and furthermore in patients prone to orthostatic syncope (Gulli et al., 2003). In this study, we found a prolonged baroreflex time delay in young diabetics using the cross-correlation method. In fact, the baroreflex time delay was the baroreflex property most impaired in our group of DM patients. The significant negative correlation between *bslope* and the baroreflex time delay imply that patients who have a low bradycardic baroreflex response also have a delayed baroreflex adaptation. We suggest that impairment of vagal influence on heart rate is responsible for this change.

Lower synchronization between heart rate and blood pressure time series might also be regarded as a marker of baroreflex impairment (Gulli et al., 2003; Pinna et al., 2002). Linear synchronization between SBP and RR intervals (or heart rate) time series is usually evaluated by cross-spectral methods, describing the linear dependence of the respective signals. Although coherence values tended to be lower in our DM group, these differences did not reach the level of statistical significance. In previous studies, a lower coherence between blood pressure and heart rate signals have been reported (Ziegler et al., 1992; Ducher et al., 1999).

NOVEL MEASURES FOR BAROREFLEX ASSESSMENT

Baroreflex functioning is traditionally analysed by linear data analysis techniques as described above. It has been proposed that those methods are not sufficient to characterize the complex interactions of blood pressure and heart rate and nonlinear measures, describing the qualitative features rather than magnitude of the signals and their interactions, are better suited (Beckers et al., 2006). Recently, new methods have been developed to assess the synchronization within cardiovascular system allowing the quantification of synchronization between SBP and RR intervals signals: the information domain synchronization index (Porta et al., 1999), the CrossSampEn method (Richman and Moorman, 2000) extended to multiple scales (CrossMSE), joint symbolic dynamics (Baumert et al., 2002) and the information-based similarity index (IBSI) developed by Yang et al (Yang et al., 2003). From these new non-linear indices, IBSI appears to be most sensitive to a decrease in heart rate and blood pressure interactions in DM. IBSI measures the similarity between two time series based on the concept of symbolic dynamics. To our knowledge, this is the first study to apply IBSI for the quantification of the similarity between SBP and RR interval time series. In the diabetic group we found higher values of IBSI (for sequence with the length of 4 beats), indicating less synchronization between blood pressure and RR intervals signals on scales corresponding to respiration related fluctuations. This finding suggests IBSI can reveal desynchronization of blood pressure and heart rate as another aspect of baroreflex impairment.

Chapter 17

CONCLUSION

Survival analyses in diabetic subjects consistently showed that impaired autonomic function is associated with an approximately doubled risk of mortality (Gerritsen et al., 2001). Autonomic function testing is essential to diagnose cardiac autonomic neuropathy, which might lead to those fatal endpoints such as sudden cardiac death (Vinik et al., 2003).

Heart rate variability (HRV) analysis is a simple, noninvasive procedure that can be conducted with minimal patient risk and low operator effort. HRV analysis is a useful tool for the diagnosis and monitoring of autonomic dysregulation. Since the cardiovascular control system is nonlinear and complex, new measures based on the theory of nonlinear dynamical systems were proposed and applied in many clinical studies. Traditionally used linear HRV parameters are usually correlated with each other and thus provide only limited additional diagnostic information. Contrary, most of the novel nonlinear measures are not significantly correlated with linear measures. Thus, complexity analysis of HRV may be a potential source for additional diagnostic information and useful for a better discrimination between different physiological and pathophysiological outcomes.

Our data on diabetic patients indicate that HRV complexity analysis provides a very sensitive tool to assess autonomic dysfunction in these patients. The magnitude and complexity of HRV were reduced in young patients with type 1 diabetes mellitus, indicating vagal dysfunction. Multiscale entropy as well as compression entropy analyses were able to detect HRV dysregulation but were not correlated with standard HRV measures. Therefore, the quantification of HRV complexity in combination with magnitude quantification might provide an improved diagnostic tool for cardioavascular autonomic neuropathy.

HRV may be easily quantified on relatively short recordings in a routine clinical setting, requiring only ECG and automated computer software, being neither cost nor labour intensive. Assessing HRV might also be suited to monitor different pharmacological and non-pharmacological treatment strategies (Maser and Lenhard, 2005). Based on our data we cannot conclude whether or not complexity measures allow a detection of autonomic dysregulation earlier than conventional HRV measures. One might speculate, however, that the loss of complexity might precede the loss of HRV magnitude, since the reduction of HRV complexity is more pronounced than the reduction in magnitude.

HRV has been traditionally used to assess cardiac autonomic dysfunction, describing the *tonic* cardiovascular neural regulation. With the availability of non-invasive beat-to-beat blood pressure measurement the assessment of *reflectory* cardiovascular control by means of baroreflex sensitivity testing has become practicable (Loimaala et al., 2003; Vinik and Ziegler, 2007). Different aspects of autonomic dysfunction can thus be diagnosed based on short noninvasive procedures while the patient is in the supine position - i.e. under conditions most suitable for routine outpatient evaluation (Frattola et al., 1997).

Young patients with diabetes mellitus show impaired bradycardic baroreflex responses, a prolonged baroreflex time delay and a decrease in the synchronization level between blood pressure and heart rate fluctuations as evaluated by the nonlinear infomation-based similarity index.

Further, the noninvasive measurement of beat-to-beat blood pressure can provide additional information on blood pressure dysregulation in DM. Multiscale entropy analysis (MSE) of spontaneous blood pressure oscillations (blood pressure variability – BPV) is able to detect subtle abnormalities in blood pressure control in young patients with DM, supporting the importance of complexity analysis. MSE is statistically independent from conventional methods and may allow a better stratification of DM patients with autonomic neuropathy than linear time domain measures.

It should be emphasized that marked differences in various cardiovascular signals properties were found in otherwise asymptomatic patients who showed normal values in the Ewing battery tests. This fact further underlines the very high sensitivity of the proposed measures.

The potentially important nonlinear measures identified in this study should be validated in larger trials – longitudinal analyses are needed to monitor the changes in HRV, BPV and baroreflex function with the progression of disease and to assess the effects of treatment. Our pilot study was conducted on a relatively small group of patients. We could not assess the relation between nonlinear measures and the severity of neuropathy in diabetics.

ACKNOWLEDGEMENTS

We acknowledge the support by project of Centre of Excellence for perinatological research No 26220120016, grant VEGA no. 1/0064/08, grant VVZ MSMT 0021622402 and by the Australian Research Council (grant# DP0663345).

REFERENCES

Angelini, L; Maestri, R; Marinazzo, D; Nitti, L; Pellicoro, M; Pinna, GD; Stramaglia, S; Tupputi, SA. Multiscale analysis of short term heart beat interval, arterial blood pressure, and instantaneous lung volume time series. *Artif. Intell. Med.*, 2007, 41: 237-50.

Batchinsky, AI; Cooke, WH; Kuusela, T; Cancio, LC. Loss of complexity characterizes the heart rate response to experimental hemorrhagic shock in swine. *Crit. Care Med.* 2007, 35: 519-25.

Baumert, M.; Walther, T; Hopfe, J; Stepan, H; Faber, R; Voss, A. Joint symbolic dynamic analysis of beat-to-beat interactions of heart rate and systolic blood pressure in normal pregnancy. *Med. Biol. Eng. Comput.*, 2002, 40: 241-45.

Baumert, M; Baier, V; Haueisen, J; Wessel, N; Meyerfeldt, U; Schirdewan, A; Voss, A. Forecasting of life threating arrhythmias using the compression entropy of heart rate. *Methods Inf. Med.*, 2004, 43: 202-26.

Baumert, M; Baier, V; Schirdewan, A; Truebner, S; Voss, A. Short- and long-term joint symbolic dynamics of heartrate and blood pressure indilated cardiomyopathy. *IEEE Trans. Biomed. Eng.*, 2005; 52: 2112-15.

Baumert, M; Lambert, G; Dawood, T; Lambert, E; Esler, M; McGrane, M; Barton, D; Sanders, P; Nalivaiko, E. Short-term heart rate variability and cardiac norepinephrine spillover in patients with depression and panic disorder. *Am. J. Physiol. Heart Circ. Physiol.*, 2009, in press.

Beckers, F; Verheyden, B; Ramaekers, D; Swynghedauw, B; Aubert, AE. Effects of autonomic blockade on non-linear cardiovascular variability indices in rats. *Clin. Exp. Pharmacol. Physiol.*, 2006, 33: 431-39.

Bernardi, L. Clinical evaluation of arterial baroreflex activity in diabetes. *Diabetes Nutr. Metab.*, 2000, 13: 331-40.

Bernardi, L; Rossi, M; Leuzzi, S; Mevio, E; Fornasari, G; Calciati, A; Orlandi, C; Fratino P. Reduction of 0.1 Hz microcirculatory fluctuations as evidence of sympathetic dysfunction in insulin-dependent diabetes. *Cardiovasc. Res.*, 1997, 34: 185-91.

Bettermann, H; Kroz, M; Girke, M; Heckmann, C. Heart rate dynamics and cardiorespiratory coordination in diabetic and breast cancer patients. *Clin. Physiol.*, 2001, 21: 411-20.

Boysen, A; Lewin, MAG; Hecker, W; Leichter, HE; Uhlemann, F. Autonomic function testing in children and adolescents with diabetes mellitus. *Pediatr. Diabetes*, 2007, 8: 261-64.

Burger, AJ; D'Elia, JA; Weinrauch, LA; Lerman, I; Gaur, A. Marked abnormalities in heart rate variability are associated with progressive deterioration of renal function in type I diabetic patients with overt nephropathy. *Int. J. Cardiol.*, 2002, 86: 281-7.

Cao, L. Practical method for determining the minimum embedding dimension of a scalar time series. *Physica D.*, 1997, 110: 43-50.

Castiglioni, P; Parati, G; Omboni, S; Mancia, G; Imholz, BPM; Wesseling, K; Di Rienzo, M. Broad-band spectral analysis of 24h continuous finger blood pressure: comparison with intra-arterial recordings. *Clin. Sci.* 1999, 97: 129-39.

Cavalcanti, S; Belardinelli, E. Modeling of cardiovascular variability using a differential delay equation. *IEEE Trans. Biomed. Eng.*, 199, 43: 982-9.

Cerutti, S; Goldberger, AL; Yamamoto, Y. Recent advances in heart rate variability signal processing and interpretation. *IEEE Trans. Biomed. Eng.*, 2006, 53: 1-3.

Chau, NP; Mestivier, D; Chanudet, X; Bauduceau, B; Gautier, D; Larroque, P. Use of runs test to assess cardiovascular autonomic function in diabetic subjects. *Diabetes Care,* 1994, 17: 146-8.

Colhoun, HM; Francis, DP; Rubens, MB; Underwood, SR; Fuller, JH. The association of heart-rate variability with cardiovascular risk factors and coronary artery calcification: a study in type 1 diabetic patients and the general population. *Diabetes Care,* 2001, 24: 1108-14.

Costa, M; Goldberger, AL; Peng, C-K. Multiscale entropy analysis of complex physiologic time series. *Phys. Rev. Lett.* 2002, 89: 068102.

Costa, M; Goldberger, AL; Peng, C-K. Multiscale entropy analysis of biological signals. *Phys. Rev. E*, 2005, 71: 021906.

Costa, MD; Peng, C-K; Goldberger, AL. Multiscale analysis of heart rate dynamics: entropy and time irreversibility measures. *Cardiovasc. Eng.,* 2008, 8: 88.

Cottin, F; Papelier, Y; Escourrou, P. Effects of exercise load and breathing frequency on heart rate and blood pressure variability during dynamic exercise. *Int. J. Sports Med.* 1999; 20: 232-8.

Dabire, H; Mestivier, D; Jarnet, J; Safar, ME; Chau, NP. Quantification of sympathetic and parasympathetic tones by nonlinear indexes in normotensive rats. *Am. J. Physiol.,* 1998, 275: H1290-7.

Ducher, M; Bertram, D; Sagnol, I; Cerutti, C; Thivolet, C; Fauvel, JP. Limits of clinical tests to screen autonomic function in diabetes type 1. *Diabetes Metab.,* 2001, 27: 545-50.

Ducher, M; Thivolet, C; Cerutti, C; Laville, M; Gustin, MP; Paultre, CZ; Abou-Amara, S; Fauvel, JP. Noninvasive exploration of cardiac autonomic neuropathy - Four reliable methods for diabetes? *Diabetes Care*, 1999, 22: 388-93.

Eckberg, DL. Physiological basis for human autonomic rhythms *Ann. Med.* 2000, 32: 341-9.

Eckberg, DL; Harkins, SW; Fritsch, JM; Musgrave, GE; Gardner, DF. Baroreflex control of plasma norepinephrine and heart period in healthy subjects and diabetic patients. *J. Clin. Invest.,* 1986, 78: 366-74.

Fraser, AM; Swinney, HL Independent coordinates for strange attractors from mutual information. *Phys. Rev. A,* 1986, 33: 1134-40.

Frattola, A; Parati, G; Gamba, P; Paleari, F; Mauri, G; DiRienzo, M; Castiglioni, P; Mancia, G. Time and frequency domain estimates of spontaneous baroreflex sensitivity provide early detection of autonomic dysfunction in diabetes mellitus. *Diabetologia,* 1997, 40: 1470-5.

Furlan, R; Porta, A; Costa, F; Tank, J; Baker, L; Schiavi, R; Robertson, D; Malliani, A; Mosqueda-Garcia R. Oscillatory patterns in sympathetic neural discharge and cardiovascular variables during orthostatic stimulus. *Circulation*, 2000, 101: 886-92.

Giudice, PL; Careddu, A; Magni, G; Quagliata, T; Pacifici, L; Carminati, P. Autonomic neuropathy in streptozotocin diabetic rats: effect of acetyl-L-carnitine. *Diabetes Res. Clin. Pract.,* 2002, 56: 173-80.

Goldberger, AL; Peng, CK; Lipsitz, LA. What is physiologic complexity and how does it change with aging and disease? *Neurobiol. Aging,* 2002, 23: 23-6.

Gonzalez, JJ; Cordero, JJ; Feria, M; Pereda, E. Detection and sources of nonlinearity in the variability of cardiac R-R and blood pressure in rats. *Am. J. Physiol.,* 2000, 279: H3040-6.

Gulli, G; Cooper, VL; Claydon, V; Hainsworth, R. Cross-spectral analysis of cardiovascular parameters whilst supine may identify subjects with poor orthostatic tolerance. *Clin. Sci.*, 2003, 105: 119-26.

Guzzetti, S; Borroni, E; Garbelli, PE; Ceriani, E; Della Bella, P; Montano, N; Cogliati, C; Somers, VK; Malliani, A; Porta, A. Symbolic dynamics of heart rate variability: a probe to investigate cardiac autonomic modulation. *Circulation*, 2005, 112: 465-70.

Hadammard, J. Les surfaces a courbures opposees et leurs lignes geodesiques. *J. Math. Pures et Appl.*, 1898, 4: 27-73.

Hayano, J; Sakakibara, Y; Yamada, A; Yamada, M; Mukai, S; Fujinami, T; Yokoyama, K; Watanabe, Y; Takata, K. Accuracy of assessment of cardiac vagal tone by heart rate variability in normal subjects. *Am. J. Cardiol.*, 1991, 67: 199-204.

Javorka, K; Javorkova, J; Petraskova, M; Tonhajzerova, I; Buchanec, J; Chroma, O. Heart rate variability and cardiovascular tests in young patients with diabetes mellitus type 1. *J. Pediatr. Endocrinol. Metab.*, 1999, 12: 423-31.

Javorka, M; Javorkova, J; Tonhajzerova, I; Javorka, K. Parasympathetic versus sympathetic control of the cardiovascular system in young patients with type 1 diabetes mellitus *Clin. Physiol. Funct. Imaging,* 2005, 25: 270-4.

Javorka, M; Trunkvalterova, Z; Tonhajzerova, I; Javorkova, J; Javorka, K; Baumert, M. Short-term heart rate complexity is reduced in patients with type 1 diabetes mellitus. *Clin. Neurophysiol.*, 2008a, 119:1071-81.

Javorka, M; Trunkvalterova, Z; Tonhajzerova, I; Lazarova, Z; Javorkova, J; Javorka K. Recurrences in heart rate dynamics are changed in patients with diabetes mellitus. *Clin. Physiol. Funct. Imaging,* 2008b, 28: 326-31.

Javorka, M; Turianikova, Z; Tonhajzerova, I; Javorka, K; Baumert, M. The effect of orthostasis on recurrence quantification analysis of heart rate and blood pressure dynamics. *Physiol. Meas.*, 2009, 30: 29-41.

Javorka, M; Zila, I; Balharek, T; Javorka, K. Heart rate recovery after exercise: relations to heart rate variability and complexity. *Braz. J. Med. Biol. Res.* 2002, 35: 991-1000.

Laitinen, T; Hartikainen, J; Niskanen, L; Geelen, G; Länsimies, E. Sympathovagal balance is major determinant of short-term blood pressure variability in healthy subjects. *Am. J. Physiol.* 1999, 276: H1245-52.

Li, M; Vitányi, P. *An introduction to Kolmogorov complexity and its applications.* 2nd edition. New York: Springer Verlag; 1997.

Liao, D; Carnethon, M; Evans, GW; Cascio, WE; Heiss, G. Lower heart rate variability is associated with the development of coronary heart disease in individuals with diabetes: the atherosclerosis risk in communities (ARIC) study. *Diabetes*, 2002, 51:3 524-31.

Loimaala, A; Huikuri, HV; Koobi, T; Rinne, M; Nenonen, A; Vuori, I. Exercise training improves baroreflex sensitivity in type 2 diabetes. *Diabetes,* 2003, 52: 1837-42.

Maestri, R; Pinna, GD; Porta, A; Balocchi, R; Sassi, R; Signorini, MG; Dudziak, M; Raczak, G. Assessing nonlinear properties of heart rate variability from short-term recordings: are these measurements reliable? *Physiol. Meas.* 2007, 28: 1067-77.

Makimattila, S; Schlenzka, A; Mantysaari, M; Bergholm, R; Summanen, P; Saar, P; Erkkila, H; Yki-Jarvinen, H. Predictors of abnormal cardiovascular autonomic function measured by frequence domain analysis of heart rate variability and conventional tests in patients with type 1 diabetes. *Diabetes Care,* 2000, 23: 1686-93.

Mancia, G; Parati, G; Pomidossi, G; Casadei, R; Dirienzo, M; Zanchetti, A. Arterial baroreflexes and blood-pressure and heart-rate variabilities in humans. *Hypertension,* 1986, 8: 147-53.

Martinmaeki, K; Rusko, H; Kooistra, L; Kettunen, J; Saalasti, S. Intraindividual validation of heart rate variability indexes to measure vagal effects on hearts. Am. J. Physiol. Heart Circ. Physiol., 2006, 290: H640-7.

Marwan, N; Romano, MC; Thiel, M; Kurths, J. Recurrence plots for the analysis of complex systems. *Phys. Rep.* 2007, 438: 237-329.

Marwan, N; Wessel, N; Meyerfeldt, A; Schirdewan, A; Kurths, J. Recurrence plot based measures of complexity and its application to heart rate variability data. *Phys. Rev. E,* 2002, 66: 026702.

Maser, RE; Lenhard, MJ. Cardiovascular autonomic neuropathy due to diabetes mellitus: clinical manifestations, consequences, and treatment. *J. Clin. Endocrinol. Metab.*, 2005, 90: 5896-903.

McNames, J; Aboy, M. Reliability and accuracy of heart rate variability metrics versus ECG segment duration. *Med. Biol. Eng. Comput.*, 2006, 44: 747-56.

Mestivier, D; Dabire, H; Chau, NP. Effects of autonomic blockers on linear and nonlinear indexes of blood pressure and heart rate in SHR. *Am. J. Physiol.,* 2001, 272: H1099-113.

Parati, G; Mancia, G; Di Rienzo, M; Castiglioni, P. Point: cardiovascular variability is/is not an index of autonomic control of circulation *J. Appl. Physiol.,* 2006, 101: 676-8; discussion 681-2.

Pecis, M; Azevedo, MJ; Moraes, RS; Ferlin, EL; Gross, JL. Autonomic dysfunction and urinary albumin excretion rate are associated with an abnormal blood pressure pattern in normotensive normoalbuminuric type 1 diabetic patients. *Diabetes Care,* 2000, 23: 989-93.

Penaz, J. Photo-electric measurement of blood pressure, volume and flow on the finger. *Digest 10th Int. Conf. Med. Biol. Eng., Dresden,* 1973: 104.

Penaz, J; Voigt, A; Teichmann, W. Contribution to the continuous indirect blood pressure measurement. *Z. Gesamte Inn. Med.,* 1976, 31: 1030-3.

Penttila, J; Helminen, A; Jartti, T; Kuusela, T; Huikuri, HV; Tulppo, MP; Scheinin, H. Effect of cardiac vagal outflow on complexity and fractal properties of heart rate dynamics. *Auton. Autacoid. Pharmacol.,* 2003, 23: 173-9.

Pincus, S. Approximate Entropy (ApEn) as a complexity measure. *Chaos,* 1995, 5: 110-7.

Pinna, GD; Maestri, R; Raczak, G; La Rovere, MT. Measuring baroreflex sensitivity from the gain function between arterial pressure and heart period. *Clin. Sci.,* 2002, 103: 81-8.

Porta, A; Baselli, G; Lombardi, F; Montano, N; Malliani, A; Cerutti, S. Conditional entropy approach for the evaluation of the coupling strength. *Biol. Cybern.,* 1999, 81: 119-29.

Porta, A; Guzzetti, S; Furlan, R; Gnecchi-Ruscone, T; Montano, N; Malliani, A. Complexity and nonlinearity in short-term heart period variability: comparison of methods based on local nonlinear prediction. *IEEE Trans. Biomed. Eng.,* 2007a, 54: 94-106.

Porta, A; Guzzetti, S; Montano, N; Furlan, R; Pagani, M; Mallian, A; Cerutti, S. Entropy, entropy rate, and pattern classification as tools to typify complexity in short heart period variability series. *IEEE Trans. Biomed. Eng.* 2001, 48: 1282-91.

Porta, A; Guzzetti, S; Montano, N; Pagani, M; Somers, V; Malliani, A; Baselli, G; Cerutti, S. Information domain analysis of cardiovascular variability signals: evaluation of regularity, synchronisation and coordination. *Med. Biol. Eng. Comput.,* 2000, 38: 180-8.

Porta, A; Tobaldin, E; Guzzetti, S; Furlan, R; Montano, N; Gnecchi-Ruscone, T. Assessment of cardiac autonomic modulation during graded head-up tilt by symbolic analysis of heart rate variability. *Am. J. Physiol. Heart Circ. Physiol.,* 2007b, 293: H702-8.

Porter, KB; O'Brien, WF; Kiefert, V; Knuppel, RA. Finapres: a noninvasive device to monitor blood pressure. *Obstet. Gynecol.,* 1991, 78: 430-3.

Raab, C; Wessel, N; Schirdewan, A; Kurths, J. Large-scale dimension densities for heart rate variability analysis. *Phys. Rev. E,* 2006, 73: 041907.

Richman, JS; Moorman, JR. Physiological time-series analysis using approximate entropy and sample entropy. *Am. J. Physiol. Heart Circ. Physiol.* 2000, 278: H2039-49.

Rollins, M; Jenkins, JG; Carson, DJ; McGlure, BG; Mitchel, RH; Imam, SZ. Power spectral analysis of the electrocardiogram in diabetic children. *Diabetologia,* 1992, 35: 452-5.

Ruiz, J; Monbaron, D; Parati, G; Perret, S; Haesler, E; Danzeisen, C; Hayoz, D. Diabetic neuropathy is a more important determinant of baroreflex sensitivity than carotid elasticity in type 2 diabetes. *Hypertension,* 2005, 46: 162-7.

Sanya, EO; Brown, CM; Dutsch, M; Zikeli, U; Neundorfer, B; Hilz, MJ. Impaired cardiovagal and vasomotor responses to baroreceptor stimulation in type II diabetes mellitus. *Eur. J. Clin. Invest.* 2003, 33: 582-8.

Schreiber, T. Interdisciplinary application of nonlinear time series methods. *Phys. Rep.* 1999, 308: 1-64.

Schroeder, EB; Chambless, LE; Liao, D; Prineas, RJ; Evans, GW; Rosamond, WD; Heiss, G. Diabetes, glucose, insulin, and heart rate variability: the Atherosclerosis Risk in Communities (ARIC) study. *Diabetes Care,* 2005, 28: 668-74.

Schroeder, EB; Chambless, LE; Liao, D; Prineas, RJ; Evans, GW; Rosamond, WD; Heiss, G. Diabetes, glucose, insulin, and heart rate variability. *Diabetes Care,* 2005, 28: 668-74.

Shannon., CE. A mathematical model of communication. *The Bell System Technical J,* 1948, 27: 379-423, 623-656.

Takalo, R; Korhonen, I; Turjanmaa, V; Majahalme, S; Tuomisto, M; Uusitalo, A. Short-term variability of blood pressure and heart rate in borderline and mildly hypertensive subjects. *Hypertension,* 1994, 23: 18-24.

Takase, B; Kitamura, H; Noritake, M; Nagase, T; Kurita, A; Ohsuzu, F; Matsuoka, T. Assessment of diabetic autonomic neuropathy using twenty-four-hour spectral analysis of heart rate variability: a comparison with the findings of the Ewing battery. *Jpn. Heart J.,* 2002, 43: 127-35.

Takens, F. Detecting strange attractors in turbulence. In: Rand, DA; Young, LS, editors. *Dynamical systems and turbulence: Lecture notes in mathematics.* Berlin: Springer-Verlag; 1981; vol. 898: 365-381.

Tarvainen, MP; Ranta-Aho, PO; Karjalainen, PA. An advanced detrending method with application to HRV analysis. *IEEE Trans. Biomed. Eng.* 2002, 49: 172-5.

Task Force of the European Society of Cardiology and the North American Society of Pacing and Electrophysiology: Heart rate variability. Standards of measurement, physiological interpretation, and clinical use. *Eur. Heart J.,* 1996,17: 354-81.

Theiler, J. Spurious dimension from correlation algorithms applied to limited time series data. *Phys. Rev. A,* 1986, 34: 2427-32.

Toyry, JP; Niskanen, LK; Lansimies, EA; Partanen, KP; Uusitupa, MI. Autonomic neuropathy predicts the development of stroke in patients with non-insulin-dependent diabetes mellitus. *Stroke,* 1996, 27: 1316-8.

Trunkvalterova, Z; Javorka, M; Tonhajzerova, I; Javorkova, J; Lazarova, Z; Javorka, K; Baumert, M. Reduced short-term complexity of heart rate and blood pressure dynamics in patients with diabetes mellitus type 1: multiscale entropy analysis. *Physiol. Meas.,* 2008, 29: 817-28.

Vinik, AI, Erbas T: Recognizing and treating diabetic autonomic neuropathy. *Cleve. Clin. J. Med.,* 2001, 68: 928-30, 932, 934-44.

Vinik, AI; Maser, RE; Mitchell, BD; Freeman, R. Diabetic autonomic neuropathy. *Diabetes Care,* 2003, 26: 1553-79.

Vinik, AI; Ziegler, D. Diabetic cardiovascular autonomic neuropathy. *Circulation,* 2007, 115: 387-97.

Virolainen, J. Use of non-invasive finger blood pressure monitoring in the estimation of aortic pressure at rest and during the Mueller manoeuvre. *Clin. Physiol.,* 1992, 12: 619-28.

Voss, A; Hnatkova, K; Wessel, N; Kurths, J; Sander, A; Schirdewan, A; Camm, AJ; Malik, M. Multiparametric analysis of heart rate variability used for risk stratification among survivors of acute myocardial infarction. *Pacing Clin. Electrophysiol.,* 1998, 21:186-92.

Voss, A; Kurths, J; Kleiner, HJ; Witt, A; Wessel, N; Saparin, P; Osterziel, KJ; Schurath, R; Dietz, R. The application of methods of non-linear dynamics for the improved and predictive recognition of patients threatened by sudden cardiac death. *Cardiovasc. Res.,* 1996, 31: 419-33.

Voss, A; Schulz, S; Schroeder, R; Baumert, M; Caminal, P. Methods derived from nonlinear dynamics for analyzing heart rate variability. *Philos. Transact. A Math. Phys. Eng. Sci.*, 2009, 367: 277-96.

Vuksanovic, V; Gal, V. Nonlinear and chaos characteristics of heart period time series: healthy aging and postural change. *Auton. Neurosci.,* 2005, 121: 94-100.

Watkins, LL; Surwit, RS; Grossman, P; Sherwood, A. Is there a glycemic threshold for impaired autonomic control? *Diabetes Care,* 2000, 23: 826-30.

Watson, AM; Hood, SG; Ramchandra, R; McAllen, RM; May, CN. Increased cardiac sympathetic nerve activity in heart failure is not due to desensitization of the arterial baroreflex. *Am. J. Physiol. Heart Circ. Physiol.*, 2007, 293, H798-804.

Webber CL. Introduction to Recurrence quantification analysis. RQA software ver. 11.1 (2007); (URL: http://homepages.luc.edu/~cwebber/).

Webber, CL; Zbilut, JP. Dynamical assessment of physiological systems and states using recurrence plot strategies. *J. Appl. Physiol.*, 1994, 76, 965-73.

Webber, CL; Zbilut, JP. Recurrence quantification analysis of nonlinear dynamical systems, Tutorials in Contemporary Nonlinear Methods for the Behavioral Science Web Book, (U.S., National Science Foundation) (2005); (URL:http://www.nsf.gov/sbe/bcs/pac/nmbs/nmbs.jsp).

Westerhof, BE; Gisolf, J; Stok, WJ; Wesseling, KH; Karemaker, JM. Time-domain cross-correlation baroreflex sensitivity: performance on the EUROBAVAR data set. *J. Hypertens.*, 2004, 22: 1371-80.

Whang, W; Bigger, JT, Jr. Comparison of the prognostic value of RR-interval variability after acute myocardial infarction in patients with versus those without diabetes mellitus. *Am. J. Cardiol.*, 2003, 92: 247-51.

Wheeler, SG; Ahroni, JH; Boyko, EJ. Prospective study of autonomic neuropathy as a predictor of mortality in patients with diabetes. *Diabetes Res. Clin. Pract.*, 2002, 58: 131-8.

Yang, ACC; Shu-Shya, H; Huey-Wen, Y; Goldberger, AL; Peng, CK. Linguistic analysis of the human heartbeat using frequency and rank order statistics. *Phys. Rev. Lett.*, 2003, 90: 108103.

Zavodna, E; Honzikova, N; Hrstkova, H; Novakova, Z; Moudr, J; Jira, M; Fiser, B. Can we detect the development of baroreflex sensitivity in humans between 11 and 20 years of age? *Can. J. Physiol. Pharmacol.*, 2006, 84: 1275-83.

Ziegler, D. Diabetic cardiovascular autonomic neuropathy: prognosis, diagnosis and treatment *Diabetes Metab. Rev.*, 1994, 10: 339-83.

Ziegler, D; Dannehl, K; Muhlen, H; Spuler, M; Gries, FA. Prevalence of cardiovascular autonomic dysfunction assessed by spectral-analysis and standard-tests of heart-rate variation in newly diagnosed IDDM patients. *Diabetes Care,* 1992, 15: 908-11.

Ziv, J; Lempel, A. An universal algorithm for sequential data compression. *IEEE Trans. Inf. Theory,* 1977, 23: 337-43.

INDEX

A

abnormalities, 5, 57, 80, 86
ACC, 93
accuracy, 89
acute, 92, 93
adaptation, 76
adjustment, 43
administration, 43
adolescents, 86
age, 5, 14, 49, 93
aging, 25, 26, 87, 92
albumin, 89
alcohol, 6
algorithm, 8, 65, 66, 93
alternative, 47
application, 3, 57, 89, 91, 92
arithmetic, 66
arrhythmia, 26, 27
arrhythmias, 85
artery, 86
assessment, 5, 18, 25, 47, 75, 76, 77, 80, 88, 93
assessment techniques, 76
assumptions, 43
asymptomatic, 80
atherosclerosis, 89

Atherosclerosis Risk in Communities, 91
atropine, 43
autocorrelation, 36, 38, 64
autonomic neuropathy, 25, 47, 75, 79, 80, 87, 89, 91, 92, 93
availability, 80
averaging, 8

B

baroreceptor, 91
battery, xi, 28, 80, 91
behavior, 37
bipolar, 6
blood glucose, 13
blood pressure, 6, 13, 19, 21, 47, 48, 49, 50, 53, 57, 61, 63, 64, 71, 75, 76, 77, 80, 85, 86, 87, 88, 89, 90, 91, 92
Body Mass Index, 6, 19
borderline, 5, 91
breast cancer, 86
breathing, 87

C

caffeine, 6
calcification, 86
cardiomyopathy, 85
cardiovascular risk, 86
cardiovascular system, 6, 77, 88
chaos, 92
cigarettes, 5
circulation, 89
classification, 10, 55, 90
clinical symptoms, 5
coding, 27
coherence, 64, 65, 69, 76
communication, 91
communities, 89
complex interactions, 77
complex systems, 89
components, 61
computation, 65
computer software, 50, 63, 80
computing, 35, 38, 66
consent, 6, 49
control group, 3, 5, 6, 13, 14, 15, 16, 18, 33, 39, 40, 41, 44, 50, 54, 55, 56, 67, 69, 70, 72, 73
coronary heart disease, 88
correlation, 3, 11, 19, 28, 51, 54, 55, 56, 64, 67, 69, 70, 73, 76, 92, 93
correlation analysis, 54
correlation coefficient, 11, 19, 51, 55, 56, 64, 67, 73
correlation function, 64
correlations, 3, 23, 24, 28, 29, 72
coupling, 90
cross-validation, 50

D

data analysis, 77
data set, 93
DBP, 49, 50, 53, 54, 55, 56, 57
death, 79, 92
decomposition, 26
depression, 85
desensitization, 93
desynchronization, 77
detection, 28, 37, 47, 57, 80, 87
determinism, 37, 39
deviation, 67
discriminant analysis, 50, 55
discrimination, 3, 57, 79
distribution, 9, 10, 27, 38, 43, 50, 67
division, 66
duration, 5, 22, 28, 29, 49, 89
dynamical system, 33, 79, 93
dynamical systems, 33, 79, 93
dysregulation, 3, 4, 25, 29, 33, 44, 47, 61, 75, 79, 80

E

elasticity, 91
electrocardiogram, 91
encoding, 65, 66
equilibrium, 6
estimators, 26
ethics, 6
excretion, 89
exercise, 87, 88

F

failure, 57
feet, 5
flow, 90
fluctuations, 7, 27, 57, 75, 77, 80, 86
Fourier, 7
fractal properties, 90
frequency distribution, 67

G

gender, 5, 14, 49
glucose, 6, 13, 19, 21, 24, 91
groups, 3, 5, 6, 13, 15, 18, 19, 22, 35, 38, 39, 41, 44, 49, 50, 53, 54, 63, 67, 69, 71, 76

H

heart, 13, 22, 79, 85, 86, 88, 89, 90, 91, 93
heart disease, 88
heart failure, 57, 92
heart rate (HR), 54
heart rate variability (HRV), 22, 79, 88
heartbeat, 93
histogram, 27
human, 87, 93
humans, 76, 89, 93
hypertension, 89, 91
hypertensive, 91

I

independence, 43
indices, 18, 28, 44, 61, 64, 65, 69, 71, 73, 77, 85
information exchange, 65
informed consent, 6, 49
inspection, 5
insulin, 86, 91, 92
interactions, 25, 77, 85
interval, 6, 7, 9, 28, 35, 37, 44, 63, 64, 67, 71, 77, 85, 93

L

labour, 80
limitation, 26
limitations, 43
linear dependence, 76
linear regression, 64
lung, 85
lyapunov exponent, 3

M

mathematics, 91
matrix, 36
mean systolic blood pressure, 50

measurement, 19, 21, 23, 24, 29, 47, 61, 64, 80, 90, 92
median, 6, 11, 19, 22, 39, 40, 41
men, 5, 19, 49
microcirculatory, 86
models, 61
modulation, 3, 26, 61, 88, 90
mortality, 79, 93
multidimensional, 35
multivariate, 25
myocardial infarction, 92, 93

N

National Science Foundation, 93
nephropathy, 86
nerve, 75, 92
neuropathy, 5, 81, 87, 91, 92
noise, 10
non-invasive, 80, 92
non-linear dynamics, 92
nonlinear systems, 3
nonparametric, 38
non-pharmacological, 80
norepinephrine, 85, 87
normal, 7, 13, 35, 80, 85, 88

O

operator, 79
order statistic, 93
orthostatic intolerance, 5
oscillations, 3, 7, 15, 21, 28, 45, 47, 50, 80
outpatient, 80

P

panic disorder, 85
parameter, 37, 44, 70
parasympathetic, 26, 27, 43, 44, 87
pathophysiological, 79
percentile, 9
pharmacological, 43, 76, 80
pharmacological treatment, 80

phase space, 35, 36, 38
physiological, 43, 58, 79, 92, 93
physiology, 3
pilot study, 81
plasma, 21, 24, 87
play, 57
poor, 88
population, 86
power, 7, 20, 25, 26, 28, 43, 50, 64
powers, 7, 15, 26
pragmatic, 9
predictability, 43, 65
prediction, 90
pregnancy, 85
probability, 8, 9, 37, 66
probands, 6, 44, 49
probe, 88
prognosis, 93
prognostic value, 93
protocol, 6, 19, 29, 35, 49, 63
pulse, 63, 71

Q

quantization, 10
quartile, 9
questionnaire, 5

R

random, 26, 37
range, 6, 11, 13, 19, 22, 35, 39, 40, 41, 65
rats, 43, 76, 85, 87
recognition, 92
recovery, 88
recurrence, 33, 36, 37, 38, 39, 43, 44, 88, 93
reflection, 37, 44
reflexes, 5
regression, 64
regular, 10, 65
regulation, 4, 29, 80
relationship, 11, 18, 29, 50
reliability, 89
renal, 86

renal function, 86
repeatability, 44
respiration, 77
respiratory, 26, 27
rhythm, 28
rhythms, 87
risk, 79, 89, 92
risk factors, 86
root-mean-square, 7, 50, 53
RQA, 33, 37, 38, 39, 41, 43, 44, 93
RR interval, 4, 6, 7, 8, 9, 28, 35, 38, 44, 49, 76, 77

S

sample, 10, 20, 22, 27, 28, 38, 65, 91
sampling, 6, 64
saturation, 35
SBP, 49, 50, 53, 54, 55, 57, 63, 64, 65, 66, 67, 71, 72, 73, 76, 77
scalar, 86
scatter, 24, 67
scatter plot, 24
SEM, 5, 21, 49, 51, 72, 73
sensation, 5
sensitivity, 57, 61, 63, 64, 65, 69, 70, 71, 75, 76, 80, 87, 89, 90, 91, 93
severity, 81
shape, 9
shock, 85
short-term, 1, 3, 4, 10, 27, 28, 47, 57, 85, 88, 89, 90, 91, 92
sign, 47, 75
signals, 3, 10, 26, 50, 54, 55, 57, 61, 64, 65, 66, 72, 76, 77, 80, 86, 90
similarity, 37, 66, 67, 72, 73, 77, 80
sinus, 26, 27, 61
sinus arrhythmia, 26, 27
skin, 5
smokers, 5
smoking, 6
software, 35, 93
spectral analysis, 6, 86, 88, 91
spectral component, 15
spectrum, 7, 64

standard deviation, 7, 8, 9, 44, 50, 53, 66
standards, 91
statistical analysis, 11
statistics, 11, 93
stimulus, 87
stochastic, 37
strange attractor, 87, 91
strategies, 80, 93
stratification, 80, 92
strength, 90
stress, 26
stroke, 92
substances, 6
survivors, 92
symbolic, 9, 10, 16, 17, 18, 22, 66, 67, 77, 85, 90
Symbolic Dynamics, 9
symbols, 9, 10, 16, 27, 65, 66
sympathetic, 7, 28, 47, 57, 75, 86, 87, 88, 92
symptoms, 5
synchronization, 61, 63, 65, 71, 72, 73, 75, 76, 77, 80
systolic blood pressure, 50, 53, 54, 55, 63, 69, 71, 85

T

thoracic, 6
threatened, 92
threshold, 36, 92
time series, 4, 7, 8, 10, 15, 21, 25, 28, 35, 43, 50, 64, 65, 66, 67, 76, 77, 85, 86, 91, 92

tolerance, 8, 36, 37, 50, 88
tonic, 80
training, 89
transfer, 65
transformation, 9, 27
turbulence, 91
type 1 diabetes, 6, 14, 15, 16, 17, 18, 22, 54, 57, 72, 75, 79, 88, 89
type 2 diabetes, 89, 91

U

unpredictability, 8
urinary, 89

V

vagal nerve, 75
validation, 89
validity, 3
variability, 7, 15, 20, 22, 23, 47, 50, 53, 55, 56, 79, 80, 85, 86, 87, 88, 89, 90, 91, 92, 93
variables, 38, 55, 87
variation, 10, 93
vasomotor, 91
vibration, 5

W

women, 5, 19, 49